Wushu!

Wushu!

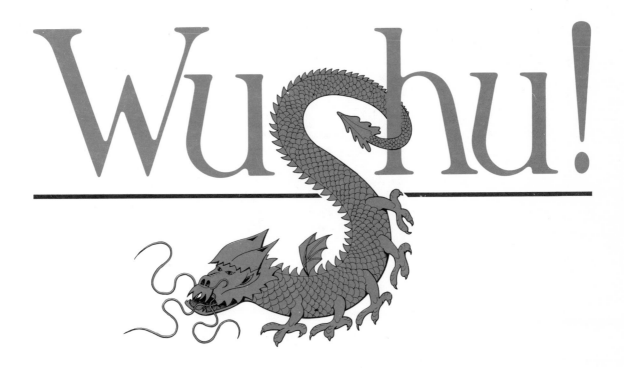

The Chinese Way To Family Health And Fitness

Introduction By
Dame Margot Fonteyn

Simon And Schuster

Material selected and translated by
TIMOTHY TUNG

from a famous series of official handbooks published in China
by The People's Sports Publishing House, Beijing

Editor **Jane Garton**
Art Editor **Ingrid Mason**
Editorial Assistant **Maxine Stait**
Illustrators **Russell Barnett**, **Nick Ward**,
The Mitchell Beazley Studio
Production **Barry Baker**

Edited and designed by
Mitchell Beazley Publishers
Mill House, 87–89 Shaftesbury Avenue, London W1V 7AD

Published in America by Simon and Schuster
A Division of Gulf and Western Corporation
Simon and Schuster Building
Rockefeller Center
1230 Avenue of the Americas
New York, New York 10020

Library of Congress Cataloging in Publication Data
Wushu! The Official Chinese Family Exercise Book
1. Martial arts
2. Exercise
3. Physical fitness – China
GV 1101. W 87   613.7   81–2739

ISBN 0–671–43887–5 Hardback edition
ISBN 0–671–42079–8 Paperback edition

Typesetting by Servis Filmsetting Ltd, Manchester
Reproduction by Dot Gradations, Chelmsford
Printed in Great Britain by Morrison & Gibb, Edinburgh
1 2 3 4 5 6 7 8 9 10

CONTENTS

INTRODUCTION

The traditional practice of Wushu is as old as Chinese culture itself, dating from the earliest Neolithic communities that first used tools and weapons to hunt for food and defend themselves. The word literally means "martial art" and, as weapons became more sophisticated, so the forms of Wushu became more varied and complex and the techniques more refined. Chiaoti, a form of wrestling that was popular amongst soldiers, and kanchiwu, an ancient dance performed with an axe and a shield, are both thought to represent stages of the early development of Wushu.

This curious mixture of a "martial art", that has become in some measure a sport and a philosophical exercise, was developed from primitive times by working people, but, as the class structure emerged within Chinese society, it was adapted by the ruling classes. They perpetuated the mythical ideas surrounding the art, claiming that anyone who had mastered Wushu was invincible in the face of physical attack. And in an attempt to protect their power, the rulers began to shroud Wushu in religious mysticism and feudal superstition, actively discouraging participation.

It was only with the founding of the People's Republic in 1949, and Chairman Mao's order to "promote physical culture and sports and build up the people's health", that every encouragement was suddenly given by the government to all aspects of Wushu – it was believed that people could play a far greater role in the construction of the new socialist state if they improved their health. Thus Wushu became the base from which to strive for intellectual, moral and physical development. And, in finding a new purpose, it acquired a sense of joy that it previously lacked.

Everywhere in China today, at dawn and dusk outside schools and factories, hospitals and shops, government offices and peasant dwellings, small children, their parents and grandparents can all be seen practising these many various forms of choreographed exercises. They are taught in schools and there are centres in every town and city, with volunteers giving free coaching to neighbourhood groups. Specialists in the art have developed new styles and techniques which are displayed at exhibitions and competitions.

Wushu, as it is now, includes a vast range of exercises that can be executed with weapons or bare-handed, with or without a partner, and they cater for all age groups. Traditionally there are two schools – the external and the internal. The external forms are sometimes hard and vigorous, involving much leaping, kicking and somersaulting. The internal school emphasizes soft, graceful, fluid movements that are similar to dancing.

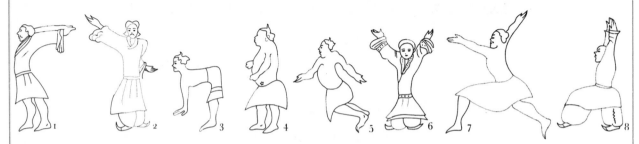

Animal Play 2,100 years ago
Animal play dates from the Han and Three Kingdoms periods when the first known physician in Chinese history, Huado (141–203), devised wuqinxi to encourage physical fitness
and improve health. Wuqinxi itself was based on even more ancient methods which mimicked the movements of animals and birds.

The earliest illustrations of animal play were unearthed a few years ago
in a general's tomb dating from the Han Dynasty (about 200 BC). The drawings of men and women exercising in animal postures are on a silk piece. Forty-four figures are depicted in different postures.

6

The internal exercises include the classic twenty-four movements in the beautifully fluid taijiquan, of which the form that creates opposing forces is somewhat akin to the isometrics that are already so popular in the West. These forms are for the elderly. In contrast, the external exercises include exercises for the new-born baby and playground exercises for school children in cities as well as those designed for country children, farmers' exercises that include charming imitations of back-breaking peasant activities like clearing up scattered grain and pounding rice with a pestle. Then there are the exercises for office workers to perform in the equivalent of our coffee break and, finally, among the external exercises, are the popular movements in imitation of animals such as the bear, tiger, monkey and crane.

The internal exercises are closer in spirit to the martial origins of Wushu, but are, in fact, gentle forms of shadow boxing and swordplay with the emphasis on fluidity. Lastly there are exercises to prevent diseases and these call for the close co-ordination of movement and breathing. They stress relaxation, tranquillity and naturalness, and they promote strength and grace in harmony.

For centuries the Chinese have had a great understanding of the mind – body relationship. To those of us in the West who are encountering the ancient wisdom of the Chinese for the first time, Wushu is among the most exciting discoveries providing, if we wish, a fascinating exercise and fitness programme for the whole family – one that subtly engages the mind and spirit in choreographic patterns of great beauty, in the swift movements of a hunter, the sophisticated co-ordinations of an athlete, the delicate balances of a gymnast, the ritual movements of a seemingly ancient and forgotten religion.

Although I was brought up in China between the ages of nine and fourteen and have throughout my life retained a deep love of the country and her people, it was not until I was older that I understood the especial cultural significance of Wushu which, of course, I was aware of every day of my childhood in China. It is, in fact, the heritage of a unique people whose civilization was already far advanced when ours was as young as a bamboo shoot, and I, for one, deeply appreciate the opportunity this book gives to master some intricacies of a movement technique that is at once classical and modern, simple and profound, absorbing and satisfying.

Margot Fonteyn

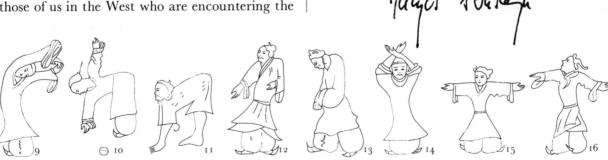

Many of the drawings have broken lines and only a few captions are legible. Researchers, however, have been able to decipher the meaning of some of them. Breathing exercises can be identified in fig 1. Figs 3 and 11 are tiger poses and fig 4 is a monkey pose. Figs 6, 7, 15 and 16 are definitely the movements of a bird. Fig 12 is a bear pose and fig 8 is possibly a deer pose.

The early Chinese also seemed to exercise with props, as can be seen from the woman body twisting in fig 10. Figs 2, 5, 9 and 14 are graceful movements that show that physical exercise had already assumed aesthetic forms in ancient times.

EXTERNAL FORMS OF EXERCISE

PRINCIPLES

The external forms of exercise are vigorous and forceful and three of the most popular with the Chinese are included here: silk exercises or baduanjin, which literally means eight section brocade; farmers' exercises or yijinjing, which literally means muscles and bones change method; and animal play or wuqinxi, which literally means five animal play. The other forms included in this section are simplified forms developed from traditional Wushu.

Silk exercises, so-called because for centuries working people have compared them to the qualities of silk brocade, call for certain essentials, as do farmers' exercises and animal play. One must be firm yet supple, and this can be achieved by relaxing muscles and nerves and then lightly tightening them when moving. This basic principle has been common to all Chinese physical exercises since the beginning of time and adherence to it relieves mental and physical fatigue.

Concentration on the lower abdomen is also important. The Chinese call this area the dantian and they compare it to a big cauldron that stores energy (qi), which can then be generated to the limbs. Concentration on this area greatly helps relaxation of body and mind and promotes blood circulation. It also helps abdominal breathing and shifts the center of gravity to the lower parts of the body which helps to steady the balance. Breathing should be natural and even throughout all these exercises and you should gradually progress to practicing abdominal breathing.

Farmers' exercises, so-called because they originated from the movements of the peasants working in the fields, can be best explained by their Chinese name yijinjing. Yi means change, jin means muscles and bones and jing means method. Together they therefore form a physical fitness program that strengthens muscles and bones. Great emphasis is put on abdominal breathing in these exercises and two different ways of doing it are explained.

Animal play exercises are so-called because the form and posture of these exercises developed from observing the movements of tiger, deer, monkey, bear and crane. It therefore involves mimicking closely each animal not only in its movement but also in its expression.

Be fierce when practicing tiger play and move in a dignified manner with piercing and shining eyes. When doing deer play imitate the relaxed manner of a deer in postures such as looking up and stretching the neck. Mimic the agility and nimbleness of a monkey in monkey play as well as its expressions in such activities as leaping, climbing and picking and offering fruits. When practicing bear play move in a firm and steady manner, but remember that the heaviness of a bear merely belies its swiftness. When practicing crane play try and imitate the arrogance of this bird.

SILK EXERCISES

The Chinese term for silk exercises is baduanjin, which literally means eight-section brocade. The four sets of exercises introduced here, each divided into eight movements, are more or less the same in principle but differ in degree of complexity. The first three sets are done in a standing position while the fourth and last is done sitting down.

To help with explanation, each movement of the first three sets is given a simple descriptive term:

Hands holding up the sky This movement relaxes the muscles and stretches the arms, legs and torso. Accompanied by deep breathing it affects the chest, abdomen and pelvis. It also helps to correct poor posture and keeps the shoulders and back straight.

Archery This movement concentrates on the chest area, but also affects shoulder and arm muscles. It helps blood circulation.

Single arm lift Stretching arms, one up, the other down, affects the liver, gall bladder, spleen and stomach and strengthens the digestive system.

Looking backward This movement involves turning the head, rolling the eyeballs and looking back as far as possible. It strengthens the neck muscles and also revitalizes the nervous system.

Head shaking and buttock swaying This movement involves using the whole body and is excellent relaxation.

Holding the toes This movement is especially good for the kidneys and waist. Bending forward and back stretches and strengthens the muscles in the waist and back, which in turn makes the kidneys and internal system firmer.

Fist play with eyes glaring The emphasis here is on glaring eyes. Exercise with an angered expression is peculiarly Chinese and combined with fist thrusting helps concentration. This movement builds up energy and strength.

Heel lifting As a conclusion heel lifting accompanied by deep breathing helps to relax the body.

THE FIRST SET

HANDS HOLDING UP THE SKY

Preparation *Stand to attention, look straight ahead and breathe through nose. Relax all joints and meditate for a few moments to gain concentration.*

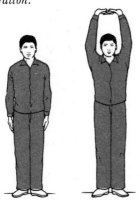

1 Slowly raise arms sideways, join hands over head, fingers interlocked, turn palms over and stretch up as though holding up the sky. At the same time lift heels off ground.
2 Lower arms and heels and return to preparation position.

Repeat exercise many times, breathe in when doing step 1; breathe out when doing step 2.

ARCHERY

Preparation *Stand to attention.*
1 Step to left and bend knees to assume a horse-riding position. Cross arms in front of chest, right arm outside, left arm inside. Then with thumb and forefinger of left hand extended and other three fingers curled, stretch left arm out to left, eyes following. At same time clench right hand and stretch to right as though pulling a bow.

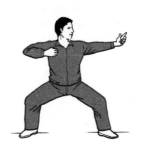

2 Return to preparation position.
3 Repeat step 1, but in opposite direction.
4 Return to preparation position. Repeat exercise many times. Breathe in when doing steps 1 and 3; breathe out when doing steps 2 and 4.

THE SINGLE ARM LIFT

Preparation *Stand straight, feet shoulder width apart, arms by side.*
1 Raise right arm over head, palm up, fingers together and pointing to ▶

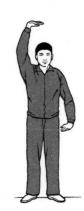

left; at same time press left hand down, palm down, fingers together and pointing straight ahead.

2 Return to preparation position.

3 Repeat step *1*, but with left arm over head.

4 Return to preparation position. Repeat exercise many times. Breathe in when doing steps *1* and *3*; breathe out when doing steps *2* and *4*.

LOOKING BACKWARD

Preparation *Stand to attention, palms tightly touching thighs.*

1 Turn head to left slowly, following movement with eyes and looking back.

2 Return to preparation position.

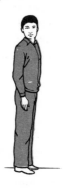

3 Turn head to right slowly, following movement with eyes and looking back.

4 Return to preparation position. Repeat exercise many times. Breathe in when doing steps *1* and *3*; breathe out when doing steps *2* and *4*.

HEAD SHAKING AND BUTTOCK SWAYING

Preparation *Bend knees to assume a horse-riding position with legs wide apart, place hands on thighs, thumbs pointing outward.*

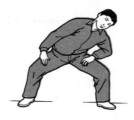

1 Bend forward from waist and rotate body toward left; at same time sway buttocks toward right.

2 Return to preparation position.

3 Repeat step *1*, but in opposite direction.

4 Return to preparation position. Repeat exercise many times. Breathe in when doing steps *1* and *3*; breathe out when doing steps *2* and *4*.

HOLDING THE TOES

Preparation *Stand to attention.*

1 Keeping knees straight and head slightly raised, bend forward slowly and hold toes, or ankles for those who cannot reach toes.

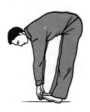

2 Return to preparation position.

3 With hands holding waist, bend back slowly.

4 Return to preparation position. Repeat exercise many times, breathing normally.

FIST PLAY WITH EYES GLARING

Preparation *Stand with legs wide apart, fists at waist and palms up. Bend knees to assume a horse-riding position.*

1 With palm down and glaring eyes following movement, stretch right fist slowly to right.

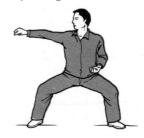

2 Return to preparation position.

3 Repeat step *1*, but to left.

4 Return to preparation position. Repeat exercise many times. Breathe out when doing steps *1* and *3*; breathe in when doing steps *2* and *4*.

HEEL LIFTING

Preparation *Stand to attention, with palms tightly touching thighs and knees straight.*

1 Hold head high and lift heels about 2 in (5 cm) off ground.

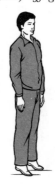

2 Lower heels to ground. Repeat exercise many times. Breathe in when doing step *1* and breathe out when doing step *2*.

THE SECOND SET

HANDS HOLDING UP THE SKY

Preparation *Stand to attention.*

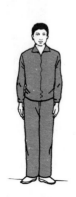

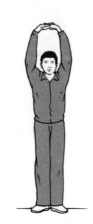

1 Relax whole body, look straight ahead, breathe normally and concentrate on lower abdomen.

2 Hold arms out to side, slowly raise them above head and interlock fingers.

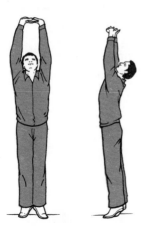

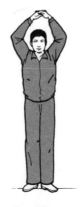

3 Keep arms straight, turn palms up and bend head back, keeping eyes on backs of hands; at the same time keep legs tightly together, lift heels, stretch body and breathe in.

4 Turn palms over and relax arms; at same time lower heels, but do not touch ground, and breathe out.
5–8 Repeat steps 3–4 twice.
9 Repeat step 3.
10 Return to preparation position and lower arms and heels.
Repeat exercise several times.

ARCHERY

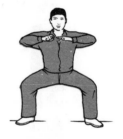

Preparation *Step to left and bend knees to assume a horse-riding position. Keep upper body straight and thighs parallel to ground. Bend arms into body at shoulder level, extend middle finger and forefinger on left hand, curl thumb and middle finger on right hand and clench all other fingers.*

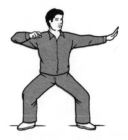

1 Push left hand to left and pull right elbow to right; keep eyes on left hand and right elbow level with shoulder. At same time expand chest, breathe in and assume position of an archer.
2 Return to preparation position, breathe out and reverse position of fingers on left and right hands.

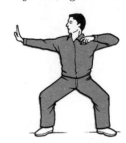

3 Repeat step 1, but in opposite direction.
4 Repeat step 2.
5–7 Repeat steps 1–3.
8 Return to preparation position.
Repeat exercise several times.

八段錦

THE SINGLE ARM LIFT

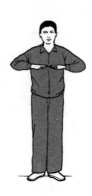 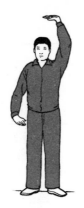 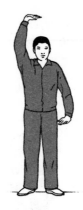

Preparation *Stand to attention. Bring hands together in front of chest, palms down, finger tips touching.*

1 Raise left hand above head, palm up, fingers pointing to the right; at same time press right hand down, point fingers straight ahead and breathe in.

2 Bend both arms until back of left hand touches top of head and right hand reaches rib cage and breathe out deeply.

3 Repeat step 1, but raise right hand and press left hand down.
4 Repeat step 2, but change hands over.
5–7 Repeat steps 1–3.
8 Return to preparation position. Repeat exercise several times. Beginners should count each step as one beat. After some practice, the movement can be speeded up by counting one beat for two steps; raise arm and return to preparation position.

LOOKING BACKWARD
Preparation *Stand to attention, chest out, stomach in, palms tightly touching thighs.*

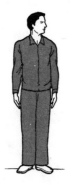 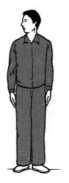 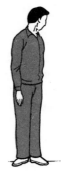

1 Without moving upper body, turn head slowly to left and look back; at same time breathe in. Turn head to front and breathe out.

2 Repeat step 1, but in opposite direction.
3–6 Repeat steps 1–2 twice.
7 Repeat step 1.
8 Return to preparation position.

Repeat exercise many times. A variation on this movement involves turning upper body with head and keeping eyes on backs of heels.

HEAD SHAKING AND BUTTOCK SWAYING

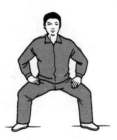 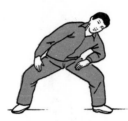

Preparation *Step to left and bend knees to assume a horse-riding position. Place hands on thighs, thumbs on outside.*

1–2 Bend upper body to left, swing head down and buttocks up to right twice; keep left arm bent and right arm straight.

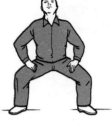 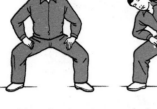

3–4 Turn head and upper body from left to back and to right.
5–6 Repeat steps 1–2, but in opposite direction.

7 Turn head and upper body from right to front and to left.
8 Stand to attention.
This exercise should be done in a continuous flow and those who are fit may repeat it three times.

HOLDING THE TOES
Preparation *Stand to attention, with knees straight and legs together.*

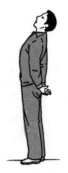 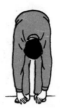

1 Hold hands behind back and bend upper body back.

2 Bend upper body forward, unclasp hands, lift over head and touch feet.
3 Bend down as far as possible and try to hold toes.
4 Repeat step 1.
5–7 Repeat step 2 three times.
8 Return to preparation position. Repeat exercise several times.

FIST PLAY WITH EYES GLARING

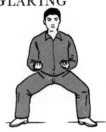

Preparation *Leap to part legs and bend knees to assume horse-riding position. Clench fists at waist, palms up, eyes glaring.*

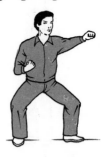

1 Thrust left fist forward with force, palm down.

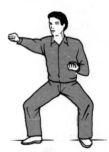

2 Draw left fist back and thrust right fist forward with force, palm down.
3 Draw right fist back and thrust left fist forward with force, palm down.
4 Repeat step 2.
5 Draw right fist back and thrust left fist to left, palm down. ▶

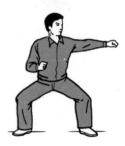

八段錦

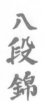

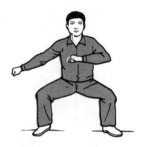

6 *Draw left fist back and thrust right fist to right, palm down.*
7 *Repeat step 5.*
8 *Drop hands and stand to attention.*
Repeat exercise many times. Variations can easily be made by thrusting right fist to left, and left fist to right.

HEEL LIFTING

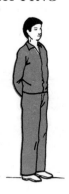

Preparation *Stand to attention, hands behind back, chest out, knees straight and legs together.*
1 *Hold head high, lift heels as high*

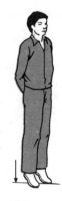

as possible and breathe in deeply.
2 *Lower heels gradually, but do not touch the ground, and breathe out.*
3–6 *Repeat steps 1–2 twice.*
7 *Repeat step 1.*
8 *Lower heels to ground and return to preparation position.*
Repeat exercise several times, then stroll around for a few moments to relax body.

TWO VARIATIONS FOR ADVANCED STUDENTS
1 Trotting *Bend knees to assume horse-riding position. Bring left hand to chest level and clench fist as*

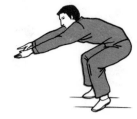

though holding reins; stretch right arm behind body and clench fist as though holding a whip. At same time, lift and lower heels in rapid succession.

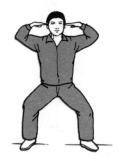

2 Galloping *Bend knees to assume horse-riding position, lean forward, stretch arms out in front; at same time lift and lower heels in rapid succession and shake whole body as though galloping at full speed.*

THE THIRD SET

HANDS HOLDING UP THE SKY

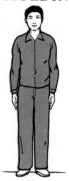

Preparation *Stand to attention.*

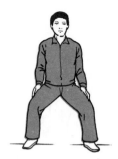

1 *Step to left and bend knees to assume a horse-riding position, arms hanging at side. Look straight ahead.*

2 *Lift hands to side of head at eye level, palms down, fingers straight.*

八段錦

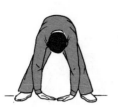

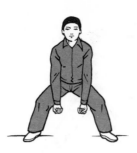

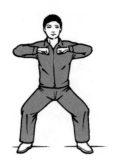

3 Bring hands down to chest level and turn fingers upright so that palms face each other with a 4–5 in (10–12 cm) space in between. Then turn palms over with finger tips of hands touching, bend forward and press down backs of hands on ground with force.

4 Turn arms so that palms face forward, clench fists and keeping arms straight, pull up body as though lifting a heavy object.

5 Bend arms and lift fists up to chest level.

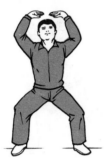

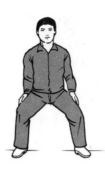

6 Open fists, palms down, turn palms out and push up with force until arms form circle; follow finger tips with eyes.

7 Drop arms but remain in horse-riding position.
8 Return to preparation position.

ARCHERY

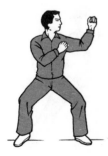

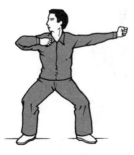

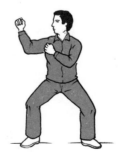

Preparation Step to left and bend knees to assume horse-riding position. Clench fists and hold left one at eye level and right one by left shoulder; keep eyes on left fist.

1 Stretch left arm to left and pull right elbow to right until both fists are at shoulder level; turn head to look at left fist and then at right.

2 Repeat preparation position, but in opposite direction.
3 Repeat step 1, but in opposite direction.
4 Return to preparation position.
5–8 Repeat steps 1–4.

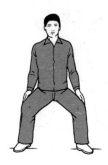

THE SINGLE ARM LIFT

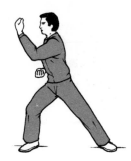

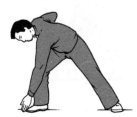

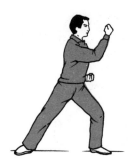

Preparation *Bend knees to assume horse-riding position, arms hanging at side and hands resting on knees. Look straight ahead.*

1 Turn body to right and straighten left leg; hold left fist up at eye level and right fist at waist, keeping eyes on left fist.

2 Bend forward and unclench fists; thrust left palm down to touch right foot and keep right hand at waist, palm up, eyes on left hand.

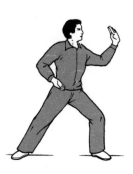

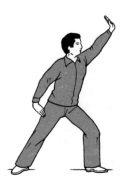

3 Turn to left and, keeping right leg straight, bend left knee; bend left arm back toward face so that fingers point at nose and eyes.

4 Push up with left hand, palm up; press down with right hand, palm down. Keep eyes on left hand.

5 Repeat step 1, but in opposite direction.

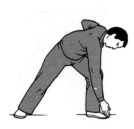

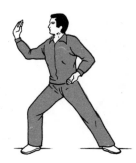

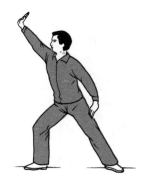

6 Repeat step 2, but in opposite direction.

7 Repeat step 3, but in opposite direction.

8 Repeat step 4, but in opposite direction.

LOOKING BACKWARD

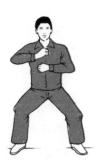

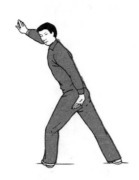

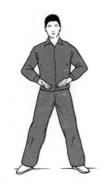

Preparation *Bend knees to assume a horse-riding position; hold right fist at chest level and left fist at stomach level, with lower fist closer to body.*

1 Turn left and, keeping right leg straight, bend left knee. At same time unclench fists and push up with right one and down with left one, eyes looking backward.

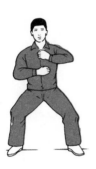

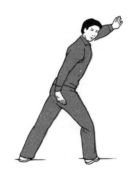

2 Turn right, return to preparation position but reverse position of fists.

3 Repeat step 1, but in opposite direction.

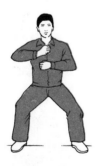

4 Repeat step 2, but in opposite direction.
5–8 Repeat steps 1–4.

HEAD SHAKING AND BUTTOCK SWAYING

八段錦

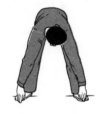

Preparation *Stand with feet apart, hands by waist, palms up, eyes looking straight ahead.*

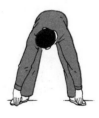

1 Bend forward without curving back and touch toes; turn head to left and buttocks to right.
2 Return to preparation position.

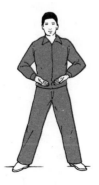

3 Repeat step 1, but turn head to right and buttocks to left.

4 Return to preparation position.
5–8 Repeat steps 1–4.

八段錦

HOLDING TOES
Preparation *Stand to attention.*

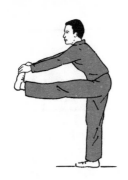

1 Keeping legs straight, lift left leg and hold toes with both hands; look straight ahead.
2 Return to preparation position.
3 Lift right leg and hold toes with both hands.
4 Return to preparation position.
5–8 Repeat steps 1–4.

FIST PLAY WITH EYES GLARING
Preparation *Stand to attention.*

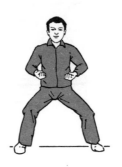

1 Step to left and bend knees to assume a horse-riding position. With eyes glaring hold fists by ribs, palms up.
2–3 Hold same position.
4 Return to preparation position. Repeat exercise several times.

HEEL LIFTING
Preparation *Stand to attention. Step to left and bend knees to assume a horse-riding position. Hold fists by chest, palms up, and look straight ahead.*

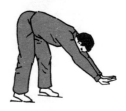

1 Lift heels high and bend forward with open palms stretched out in front. Do not curve back, follow hands with eyes.
2 Return to preparation position.
3–8 Repeat steps 1–2 three times.

THE FOURTH SET

Do these exercises sitting down in bed in the morning or before going to sleep at night.

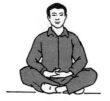

Preparation *Sit cross-legged in a half-lotus position, shoulders relaxed. Hold hands in front of abdomen, breathe normally and concentrate on lower abdomen.*

HUGGING THE HEAD
1 Hold hands behind head, fingers interlocked. Lean head backward,

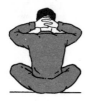

breathe in, look up; press hands forward, breathe out, look down. Repeat many times.

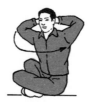

2 Turn head to left, breathe in; press hands to right, breathe out. Follow direction head is turning with eyes.
3 Repeat step 2, but in opposite direction.
Repeat exercise many times.

Physical effects Strengthens neck muscles and quickens blood circulation in head and neck. Those with high blood pressure may want to omit this exercise.

ROLLING THE HEAD
1 Relax all muscles, rest hands on knees and try not to move shoulders and arms.

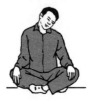

2 Roll head in half-circle from left to right a few times, and then from right to left a few times. Contract

and expand abdomen in rhythm with rolling head. Neck muscles should also be relaxed and move with movement of waist.

Physical effects Such movements of waist, head and neck have positive effects on muscles of upper body. They also activate internal organs and help blood circulation.

HOLDING UP THE SKY

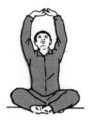

1 Join hands over head with fingers interlocked, turn palms over and push up with force; extend arms and straighten elbows, with torso stretched and stomach pulled in. At same time breathe in.

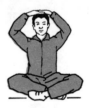

2 Relax, bringing hands down to touch top of head, and breathe out. Repeat exercise many times.

Physical effects Strengthens muscles in arms and prevents hemorrhoids.

REACHING FOR TOES
1 Remain seated and extend legs, keeping knees straight and together.
2 Bend forward as far as possible

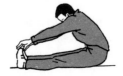

and touch toes. Keep back straight and arms stretched, and try and get forehead down as close as possible to knees.

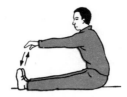

3 Bounce back quickly and repeat up and down movement of arms and torso many times.

Physical effects Strengthens kidneys and muscles in waist, back and legs.

WHEELING THE ARMS

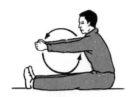

1 Remain seated with legs stretched, extend fists and move them into body and out again in a wheel-like motion. Repeat in opposite direction.

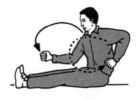

2 Repeat wheel-like motion, but alternate forward and backward movement with alternate arms. Sway head and shoulders in rhythm with movement of arms.

Physical effects Prevents shoulder and elbow ailments.

DRAWING THE BOW
1 Return to half-lotus position, bring hands up to chest then extend

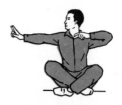

right hand, forefinger and middle finger pointing up to the right, eyes following, and pull left elbow to left with force. Expand chest once and return to half-lotus position.
2 Repeat step 1, but extend left hand and pull right elbow to right. Repeat exercise many times.

Physical effects Strengthens muscles in chest and back, increases lung capacity and improves breathing.

CRISSCROSS FIST PLAY

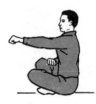

1 Thrust fists forward, left fist first, right fist second.
2 Thrust fists sideways, left fist to left, right fist to right.
3 Thrust fists crossways, left fist to right, right fist to left. Repeat exercise many times.

Physical effects Strengthens muscles in shoulders and increases nimbleness of arms.

TAPPING THE WHOLE BODY
Clench fists loosely and tap whole body, starting with waist and back and going on to chest, stomach, shoulders, neck, arms and legs.

Physical effects Loosens up and relaxes muscles and nerves in all parts of body.

嬰兒保健操

First-Year Exercises

Here are three sets of exercises for babies between the ages of two months and one and a half years. Children are greatly helped in their physical and intellectual development if they start a physical fitness program at an early age. To get the best results the following rules must be adhered to.

1 Do exercises before feeding time.
2 Do exercises in surroundings familiar to baby.
3 Make sure that bed or table is of a suitable height.
4 A kindly, patient manner must be maintained. Coax child constantly with soft simple words and make sure that the guiding movements are gentle.
5 Consistency and regularity in exercising ensure the best results.
6 Do not exercise for too long; 10–20 minutes is about right.

Passive Exercises

These exercises are for two- to six-month-old babies. Babies of between two and four months should only perform the first four exercises and the last one. Babies of between four and six months may do all eight exercises.

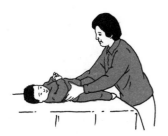

Prepare baby for exercises by placing him on bed or table and gently massaging him from chest down to abdomen and talking in a gentle tone.

Chest Exercise

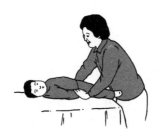

Preparation *Keep baby's arms straight, hold wrists and let him grip your thumbs.*

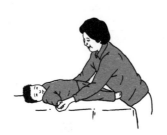

1 Spread baby's arms out to sides with palms up.

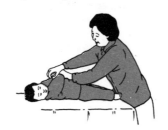

2 Bring baby's arms in and across chest and gently press his abdomen.
3 Repeat step 1.
4 Return to preparation position.
5–8 Repeat steps 1–4.
Repeat exercise twice, each time to a count of eight.

Points to remember
● *When spreading out baby's arms, be firm.*
● *When bringing baby's arms in and across chest, be gentle.*

Stretching Arms
Preparation *Keep baby's arms straight, hold wrists and let him grip your thumbs.*

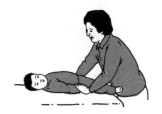

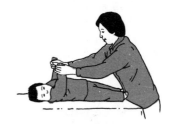

1 Pull baby's arms straight up, palms facing each other.

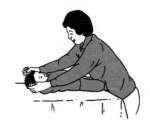

2 Place baby's arms on bed, hands above head.
3 Repeat step 1.
4 Return to preparation position.
5–8 Repeat steps 1–4.
Repeat exercise twice, each time to a count of eight.

Points to remember
● *Be gentle throughout exercise.*
●*When raising arms, make sure they are shoulder-width apart.*

20

BENDING LEGS

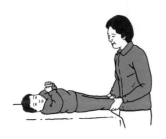

Preparation Hold baby's ankles, keeping legs straight.

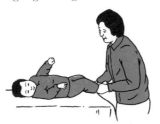

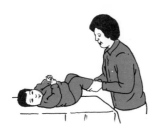

1 Bend baby's knees.
2 Straighten baby's legs.
3–8 Repeat steps 1–2 three times.
Repeat exercise twice, each time to a count of eight.

Points to remember
● When bending knees, be firm so that knees touch abdomen.
● Straighten legs gently.

RAISING LEGS

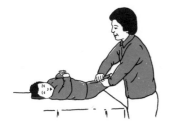

Preparation Hold baby's knees and press knee caps gently down with four fingers of each hand.

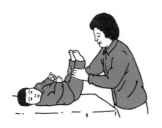

1 Lift baby's legs straight up at a 90-degree angle.
2 Return to preparation position.
3 Repeat step 1.
4 Return to preparation position.
5–8 Repeat steps 1–4.
Repeat exercise twice, each time to a count of eight.

Points to remember
● When raising baby's legs, do not lift buttocks up and be gentle.

ROTATING SHOULDERS

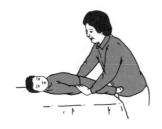

Preparation Keep baby's arms straight, hold wrists and let him grip your thumbs.
1 Rotate baby's arms outward from chest.

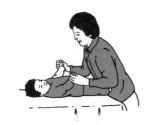

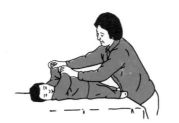

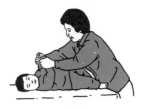

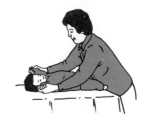

2 Return to preparation position.
3 Rotate baby's arms inward from chest.
4 Return to preparation position.
5–8 Repeat steps 1–4.
Repeat exercise twice, each time to a count of eight.

Points to remember
● Rotate arms slowly and gently.
● Do not force baby to exercise.

BENDING BACK

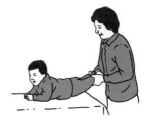

Preparation Place baby on stomach, arms out in front and elbows supporting torso; hold baby's ankles.

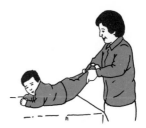

1 Lift baby's legs gently but do not move chest. ▶

嬰兒保健操

2 *Return to preparation position.*
3 *Lift baby's upper body up by elbows but do not raise abdomen off platform.*

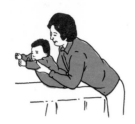

4 *Return to preparation position.*
5–8 *Repeat steps 1–4.*
Repeat exercise twice, each time to a count of eight.

Points to remember
● *Do not lift baby's legs or upper body too high.*
● *Maintain an angle at waist of no more than 45 degrees.*
● *If baby resists by twisting body, do not do this exercise.*

TURNING OVER

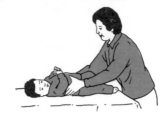

Preparation *Rest baby on bed or table.*
1 *With one hand at baby's ankles and other at bottom turn baby over to lie on stomach and make baby lift head and shoulders a little.*

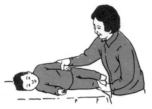

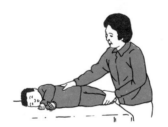

2 *Change hands and reverse movement, turning baby over to lie on his back by first lifting chest.*
3–4 *Repeat steps 1–2, but in opposite direction.*
5–8 *Repeat steps 1–4.*
Repeat exercise twice, each time to a count of eight.

Points to remember
● *Move slowly and gently.*
● *This exercise prepares baby to crawl, sit and stand.*

RELAXING
Finish off exercises by gently swinging baby's arms and legs and letting him lie on table or bed for a few moments of free movement. This should relax his muscles and mind and he should soon fall asleep.

INTER-ACTIVE EXERCISES

These exercises are for six- to twelve-month-old babies. Babies of between six and nine months should only perform the first five exercises and the last one. Babies of between nine and twelve months may do all nine exercises.

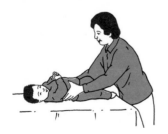

Prepare baby by placing him on bed or table and gently massaging him

from waist down to abdomen and talking gently to him.

CHEST EXERCISE

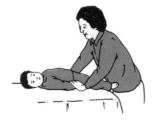

Preparation *Keep baby's arms straight, hold wrists and let him grip your thumbs.*
1 *Spread baby's arms out to side with palms up.*

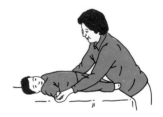

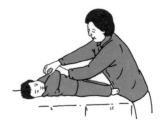

2 *Bring baby's arms in and across chest and gently press his abdomen.*
3 *Repeat step 1.*

4 *Return to preparation position.*
5–8 *Repeat steps 1–4.*
Repeat exercise twice, each time to a count of eight.

Points to remember
● *When spreading out baby's arms, be firm.*
● *When bringing baby's arms in and across chest, be gentle.*

STRETCHING ARMS

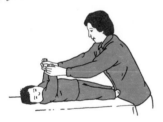

Preparation *Keep baby's arms straight, hold wrists and let him grip your thumbs.*

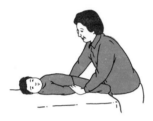

1 *Pull baby's arms straight up, palms facing each other.*

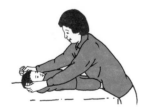

2 *Place baby's arms on bed, hands above head.*
3 *Repeat step 1.*
4 *Return to preparation position.*
5–8 *Repeat steps 1–4.*
Repeat exercise twice, each time to a count of eight.

Points to remember
● *Be gentle throughout exercise.*
● *When lifting baby's arms, make sure they are shoulder-width apart.*

BENDING LEGS.

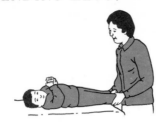

Preparation *Hold baby's ankles, keeping legs straight.*

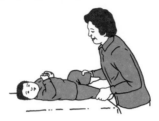

1 *Bend baby's left knee.*
2 *Return to preparation position.*

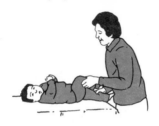

3 *Bend baby's right knee.*
4 *Return to preparation position.*
5–8 *Repeat steps 1–4.*
Repeat exercise twice, each time to a count of eight.

Points to remember
● *Bend baby's knees one at a time and keep other leg straight.*
● *Touch abdomen with knee.*

SITTING UP
For six- to nine-month-old babies

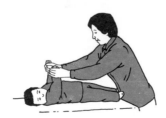

Preparation *Lay baby on back and hold hands straight up.*

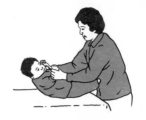

1 *Gently pull baby up to sitting position.*
2 *Return to preparation position.*
3 *Repeat step 1.*
4 *Return to preparation position.*
5–8 *Repeat steps 1–4.*
Repeat exercise twice, each time to a count of eight.

For nine- to twelve-month-old babies

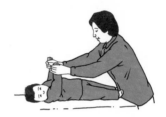

Preparation *Lay baby on back and hold hands straight up.*

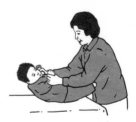

1 *Pull baby up to sitting position.*

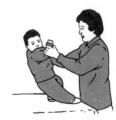

2 *Pull baby up from sitting position to standing position.*
3 *Return baby to sitting position.*
4 *Return to preparation position.*
5–8 *Repeat steps 1–4.*
Repeat exercise twice, each time to a count of eight. ▶

嬰兒保健操

嬰兒保健操

Points to remember
● *Hold baby's elbows instead of wrists if necessary.*
● *Let baby move naturally as much as possible.*

BENDING BACK

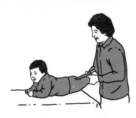

Preparation *Place baby on stomach, arms out in front and elbows supporting torso; hold baby's ankles.*

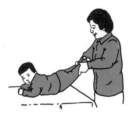

1 Lift baby's legs gently but do not move chest.
2 Return to preparation position.

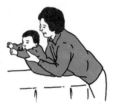

3 Lift baby's upper body up by elbows but do not raise abdomen off platform.
4 Return to preparation position.
5–8 Repeat steps 1–4.
Repeat exercise twice, each time to a count of eight.

Points to remember
● *Do not lift baby's legs or upper body too high.*
● *Maintain an angle at waist of no more than 45 degrees.*
● *If baby resists by twisting body, do not do this exercise.*

BENDING DOWN AND STANDING UP

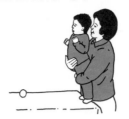

Preparation *Stand baby up and place toy in front of baby. Put one arm round abdomen and other round knees.*
1 Tighten grip round baby and let him bend forward to pick up toy.

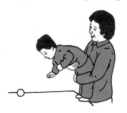

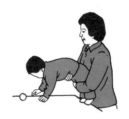

2 Return to preparation position.
3–8 Repeat steps 1–2 three times. Repeat exercise twice, each time to a count of eight.

Points to remember
● *This exercise is meant to induce baby to bend forward and straighten up on his own accord.*

RISING AND SQUATTING

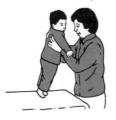

Preparation *Stand baby up, facing you, and put hands under arms.*

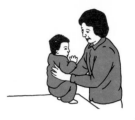

1 Lower baby to squatting position.
2 Return to preparation position.
3–8 Repeat steps 1–2 three times. Repeat exercise twice, each time to a count of eight.

Points to remember
● *Do not force baby, but try and induce him to squat and rise on his own.*
● *After baby has mastered movement hold him by wrists.*

JUMPING

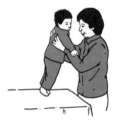

Preparation *Stand baby up, facing you, and put hands under baby's arms.*

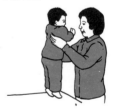

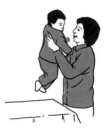

1 Hold baby under arms and encourage him gently to jump up and down.

2 Return to preparation position.
3–8 Repeat steps 1–2 three times. Repeat exercise twice, each time to a count of eight.

Points to remember
● *Movements must be light and gentle.*
● *Let baby's toes touch down gently.*
● *Encourage baby to jump on own initiative and avoid lifting him completely.*

RELAXING
Finish off exercises by gently swinging baby's arms and legs and letting him lie on table or bed for a few moments of free movement. This should relax his muscles and mind and he should soon fall asleep.

嬰兒保健操

DOUBLE POLE EXERCISES

These exercises are for one- to one-and-a-half-year-old babies. They are simple, safe, easy to learn and fun to do. Use two straight, wood, bamboo or plastic poles as props and make sure that they are thin enough for child's hands to get a grip on. Two adults are required to hold the poles. The preparation position is identical for each exercise and is therefore explained only once.

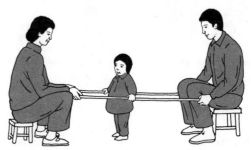

Preparation *Adults sit on small stools facing each other, holding* both ends of poles. Child stands between poles, holding onto them.*

ARM SWINGING
Repeat preparation position.

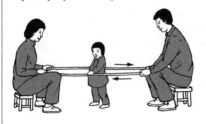

Adults move poles backward and forward alternately. Make movement gentle and rhythmic so that child's arms swing automatically with poles. Child's body should be completely relaxed.

STRETCHING
Repeat preparation position.
1 Adults move poles out to side so

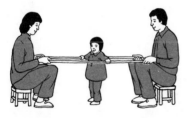

that child's arms are stretched horizontally.
2 Adults lift poles gently so that child's arms are raised over head.

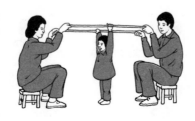

3 Adults lower poles so that child's arms are again stretched out horizontally.
4 Return to preparation position.

Points to remember
● *Do movements in a gentle and continuous flow.*
● *Child's arms must be straight and adults must not move poles too much out to side or too high so as to cause child discomfort.*

BENDING SIDEWAYS
Repeat preparation position.
1 Adults move poles out to sides so that child's arms are stretched horizontally.
2 Adults lift one pole gently up and lower other pole alternately so that child bends upper body first to left then to right, arms moving with poles.

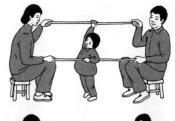

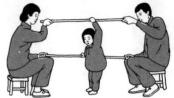

Points to remember
● *Child's upper body should not lean forward, legs should not bend, and extent of bending should increase.*

婴儿保健操

SQUATTING

Repeat preparation position.

1 Start by doing stretching exercise once, then slowly lower poles so that child lowers torso to full squat position.

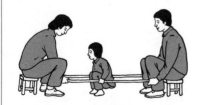

2 Adults lift poles so that child stands up and returns to position where arms are stretched out to side. Repeat exercise several times.

Points to remember
● *When lifting and lowering poles, movements should be gentle and in rhythm.*
● *Lower poles as far as possible so that child reaches a full squat with knees together and buttocks below knees.*

STEPPING FORWARD AND BACKWARD

Repeat preparation position.

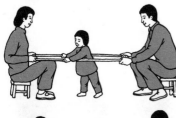

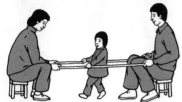

Adults move poles slowly forward and backward so that child steps forward and backward.

Points to remember
● *Make sure that child keeps balance.*

REACHING HIGH

Repeat preparation position.

1 Adults place one pole on one side of child just below bottom rib and lift other pole high so that child's other arm is raised high and straight. Lift pole high enough so that child's upper body and one arm are fully extended.

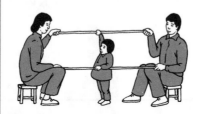

2 Return to preparation position and repeat step 1 on opposite side.

Points to remember
● *Child must keep torso straight and not bend toward either side.*

JUMPING

Repeat preparation position.
1 Adults lift poles and rest them under child's arms.

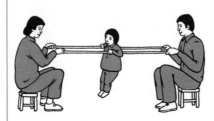

2 Use encouraging words to induce child to jump up and down as you gently lower and raise poles.

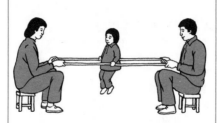

3 After short period of time child should be confident enough to jump up and down without having to lean arms on poles.

ROWING

Repeat preparation position.

1 Adults use only one pole and hold it at either end with child holding it in middle with both hands.

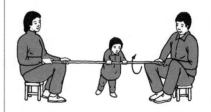

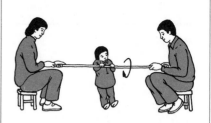

2 Turn pole round so that child's arms and upper body move with pole as though rowing a boat.

Points to remember
● *Child must not move feet.*
● *Backward and forward movement of upper body must be steady so that child is able to balance.*

幼儿保健操
PLAYGROUND EXERCISES

This series of children's exercises was developed from the basic movements of wushu. It is divided into eight sets each consisting of four positions, beginning and ending with preparation position. There are therefore only three main movements in each set. Repeat each set about twice to four times, each time to a count of eight.

The exercises are especially designed for children between the ages of three and six years. The first four sets are for three- and four-year-olds while five-year-olds can proceed to the sixth set and six-year-olds to the eighth set.

It is helpful for someone to count the beats aloud: "one, two, three, four" and so on.

THE FIRST SET

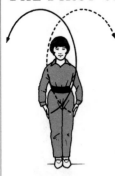 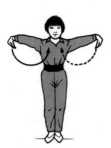 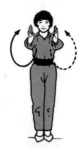 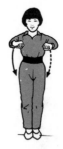 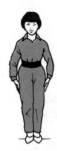

Preparation *Stand to attention with arms by side, elbows slightly bent, chest out and stomach in.*
1 Cross arms in front of chest, raise them above head and stretch them to side, hands hooked down; wrists should be slightly higher than shoulder level.

2 Lower arms and push straight forward from waist level with open hands, palms facing each other; arms should be shoulder-level high and shoulder-width apart.

3 Bring hands back to waist and stretch arms, first to side and then to front. Clench fists and bend elbows at shoulder level.
4 Return to preparation position.
5–8 Repeat steps 1–4.

THE SECOND SET

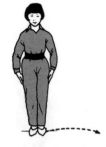 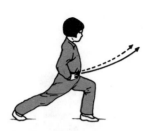 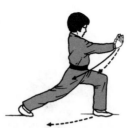 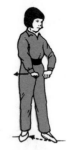 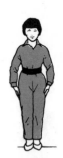

Preparation *Stand to attention with arms by side, elbows slightly bent, chest out and stomach in.*
1 With hands at waist step to left and, keeping right leg straight, bend left leg and turn body to left.

2 Push forward with open palms, arms at shoulder level.
3 Put weight on right foot and turn body toward right. Draw left foot in, pointing toes to ground; at same time bring arms in at chest level and

press down with clenched fists.
4 Return to preparation position.
5–8 Repeat steps 1–4, but in opposite direction.

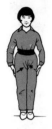

THE THIRD SET

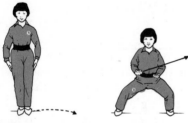 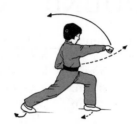 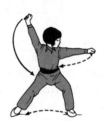 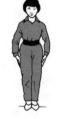

Preparation *Stand to attention with arms by side, elbows slightly bent, chest out and stomach in.*
1 Step to left, toes pointing forward. Bend knees to assume horse-riding position, chest out, stomach in, and in a continuous

motion cross arms in front, lift them above head, stretch them to side in a curve and return them to waist with clenched fists, palms up.
2 Turn to left and, keeping right leg straight, bend left leg. Thrust right fist forward with palm down.

3 Turn to right and return to horse-riding position. At same time lift right arm up and thrust left fist to left.
4 Return to preparation position.
5–8 Repeat steps 1–4, but in opposite direction.

THE FOURTH SET

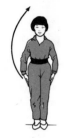 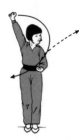 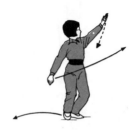 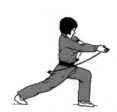 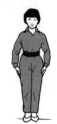

Preparation *Stand to attention with arms by side, elbows slightly bent, chest out and stomach in.*
1 Lift right fist straight up, hold left fist at waist, palm up and turn head to left.
2 Leap to left, follow with right foot, lift right heel off ground and

bend both knees slightly. At same time raise left arm, palm up, and lower right arm, pressing down fist (fists must first pass each other in front of chest).
3 Stretch right leg to right and turn body to left, keeping left leg bent and right leg straight. At same time

thrust right hand forward (in direction you are facing now) and place left hand on right elbow.
4 Return to preparation position.
5–8 Repeat steps 1–4, but in opposite direction.

THE FIFTH SET

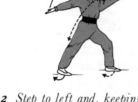 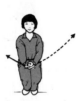 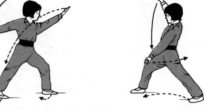 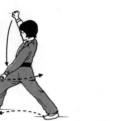 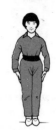

Preparation *Stand to attention with arms by side, elbows slightly bent, chest out and stomach in.*
1 Keeping knees together, squat; at same time stretch arms in front and throw left fist into right palm.

2 Step to left and, keeping right leg straight, bend left leg. At same time spread arms to side with palms up and keep eyes on left hand.
3 Turn to right and, keeping left leg straight, bend right leg. At same

time place left fist on right knee, palm facing out, and lift right fist straight up.
4 Return to preparation position.
5–8 Repeat steps 1–4, but in opposite direction.

PLAYGROUND EXERCISES

THE SIXTH SET

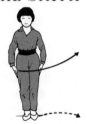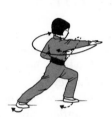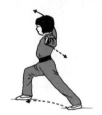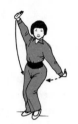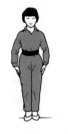

Preparation *Stand to attention with arms by side, elbows slightly bent, chest out and stomach in.*
1 Stretch right leg to right, turn body to left and with right leg straight, bend left leg. At same time thrust right hand forward (in direction you are facing now) and

keep left hand at waist, palm up.
2 Turn to right and, with left leg straight, bend right leg. At same time pass left hand above right elbow and spread arms to side, palms facing forward.
3 With right leg still bent bring left foot close to right foot, left heel

off ground; at same time raise right arm, palm up, and stretch left arm toward back, wrist hooked up.
4 Return to preparation position.
5–8 Repeat steps 1–4, but in opposite direction.

THE SEVENTH SET

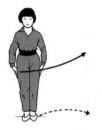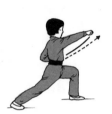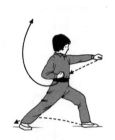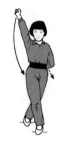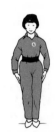

Preparation *Stand to attention with arms by side, elbows slightly bent, chest out and stomach in.*
1 Step to left, turn body to left and, keeping right leg straight, bend left leg; at same time thrust right fist forward (in direction you are facing

now), palm down, and hold left fist at waist, palm up.
2 Thrust left fist forward and bring right fist to waist.
3 Put weight on right foot and draw left foot behind with only toes touching ground; at same time push

right fist down to right and then lift it up in a curve; rest left fist on small of back.
4 Return to preparation position.
5–8 Repeat steps 1–4, but in opposite direction.

THE EIGHTH SET

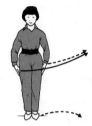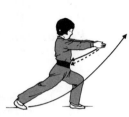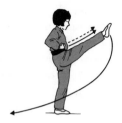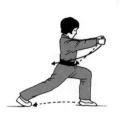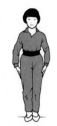

Preparation *Stand to attention with arms by side, elbows slightly bent, chest out and stomach in.*
1 Step to left, turn body to left, and keeping right leg straight, bend left leg; at same time raise arms to shoulder level and clap hands.

2 Lower hands to waist and clench fists, palms up; at same time, keeping legs straight, kick up with right foot.
3 Lower right foot to same spot and return to position with one leg bent and one leg straight, as in step 1.

At same time thrust fists forward (in direction you are facing now), palms facing each other.
4 Return to preparation position.
5–8 Repeat steps 1–4, but in opposite direction.

FARMERS' EXERCISES

Known as yijinjing these are among China's most popular exercises and are supposed to have originated from the movements of peasants working in the fields. Three sets are included here; the first and the third have 10 movements while the second has 12. All are simplified versions of ancient originals and are independent of each other. They can therefore be done in any order, and one can practice all or any of the three sets according to one's physical condition.

Breathing using abdominal muscles is an integral part of yijinjing, and there are two ways of doing this, both of which help to strengthen internal organs. One can either breathe in with abdomen contracted and chest expanded, or breathe in with abdomen expanded and chest pulled in. The second method is more natural, but advanced students may wish to try the first method. Always breathe in slowly and retain air while expanding the abdomen by lowering the diaphragm.

THE FIRST SET

This set is essentially a collection of simple breathing exercises. Beginners should repeat each of the 10 movements eight or nine times while later the number can be increased to 30 or 40.

BREATHING WITH CLENCHED FISTS
Preparation *Stand with feet shoulder-width apart; clench fists and point thumbs toward thighs. Relax shoulders and chest, look straight ahead, mouth closed, tongue touching palate and concentrate on area of lower abdomen.*

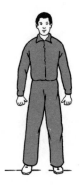

Breathe, using abdominal muscles, expanding abdomen when breathing in and tightening clenched fists when breathing out.

BREATHING WITH HANDS PRESSING DOWN
Preparation *Stand with feet shoulder-width apart, arms hanging by side, palms facing down and fingers pointing out.*

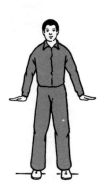

Keeping legs straight, breathe using abdominal muscles and press down with open palms. Expand abdomen when breathing in, stretch arms down when breathing out and at same time bend fingers up as much as possible so as to cause whole body to tense up.

BREATHING WITH PALMS UP
Preparation *Stand with feet shoulder-width apart. Stretch arms to side at shoulder level, palms up.*

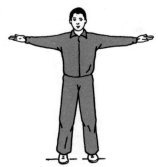

Breathe in to expand stomach and breathe out, stretching arms and hands out as much as possible as though carrying heavy objects.

BREATHING WITH PALMS PUSHING OUT
Preparation *Stand with feet shoulder-width apart. Stretch arms*

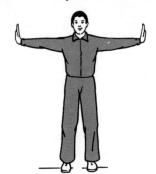

out to side at shoulder level and bend wrists so that hands are upright with open palms facing out.

Breathe in to expand stomach and breathe out while pushing hard with open palms until whole body becomes tense. Bend fingers toward head as much as possible.

BREATHING WITH PALMS TOGETHER AND APART

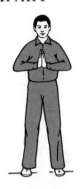

Preparation Stand with feet shoulder-width apart. Hold palms together with thumbs touching chest and elbows facing out.

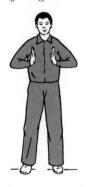

Breathe in and slowly move palms away from each other, sliding thumbs along chest. As you breathe out move palms slowly back together. Keep breathing slowly and evenly, but use enough force so as to tense whole body.

BREATHING WITH ONE ARM UP

Preparation Step to left, bend left leg, keep right leg straight and upper body upright. Raise left hand, palm up and drop right hand, palm facing inward, and point to ground.

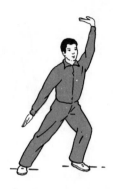

Breathe in and push left hand up and pull right arm down, tensing whole body as you do so. Relax as you breathe out.

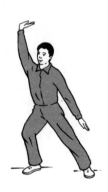

Repeat movement with right hand up and left hand down.

BREATHING WHILE SQUATTING

Preparation Stand at ease, with legs apart at a distance slightly wider than shoulder width.

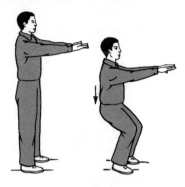

Stretch arms out in front, palms up. Turn palms over and squat down slowly until thighs are parallel to ground, keeping upper body straight.

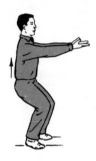

Turn palms up and lift body slowly from squatting position.

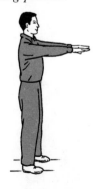

Turn palms over, ready to squat again. Repeat exercise many times, breathing in·deeply when palms are facing up.

Physical effects When done regularly strengthens kidneys and waist.

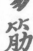

BREATHING IN A HALF-SQUATTING POSITION

Preparation *Stand at ease, legs apart at a distance slightly wider than shoulder width. Place hands behind back, clench right fist and hold it with left hand.*

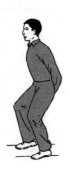

Bend knees slightly in a half-squatting position and breathe with abdominal muscles, expanding abdomen when breathing in and contracting abdomen as much as possible when breathing out.

Physical effects When done regularly helps bring down high blood pressure and strengthens leg muscles.

BREATHING WHILE BENDING DOWN

Preparation *Stand at ease with feet shoulder-width apart.*

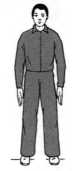
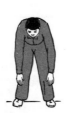

Bend upper body slowly forward at a 90-degree angle, arms hanging loose, shoulders relaxed, palms facing in and fingers pointing down. Breathe out when bending down; breathe in when straightening up.

Physical effects Helps eliminate fat in abdomen and relieves backache.

BREATHING WITH A BACKWARD TWIST

Preparation *Stand at ease. Step to left, bend left leg and keep right leg straight. Twist body to left, placing left hand on small of back, palm facing out; curve right hand*

and hold it a fist's distance away from forehead, palm facing outward. Keep eyes on right heel, which should remain on ground.

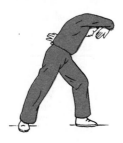

Breath using abdominal muscles; tense body twisting when breathing in and imagine that you are lowering weight to right heel when breathing out.

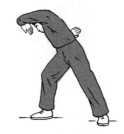

Repeat exercise, but to the right.

Physical effects Helps prevent and relieve backache.

THE SECOND SET

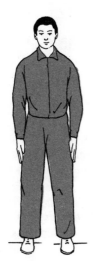

The 12 movements in this set were developed from the movements of farmers working in the fields. The preparation position is identical for each movement and is therefore explained only once.

Preparation *Stand at ease with feet shoulder-width apart, look straight ahead, breathe normally and concentrate on lower abdomen.*

HUSKING GRAIN WITH MORTAR AND PESTLE

Repeat preparation position.

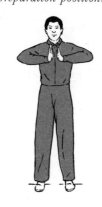

Bring hands up to chest, elbows facing out, palms facing each other about 3 in (8 cm) apart and fingers pointing up. Bring palms together and breathe 10–20 times. When breathing in, hold palms tightly together but bend fingers of both hands out; when breathing out, relax forearms.

CARRYING GRAIN WITH SHOULDER POLE

Repeat preparation position. Bring hands up to chest and stretch arms slowly out to side with open, upright palms facing out.

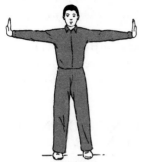

Breathe 10–20 times in this position. When breathing in expand chest and press arms back; when breathing out bend fingers in and press palms out.

WINNOWING GRAIN

Repeat preparation position. Raise arms above head, elbows straight, palms up, fingers pointing toward each other; stretch whole body as much as possible.

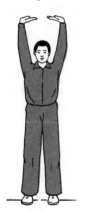

Breathe 10–20 times in this position. Breathe through nose and push up palms firmly; breathe out through mouth and relax arms.

LIFTING GRAIN ON ONE SHOULDER

Repeat preparation position. Raise right hand above head, palm down, keeping eyes on palm. Place left hand on small of back.

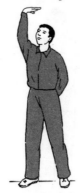

Breathe 10–20 times in this position. When breathing in, stretch head upward and shoulders back; when breathing out, relax body. Repeat exercise, but with left hand up and right hand down.

PUSHING SACKS TO PROP UP GRAIN

Repeat preparation position. Stand with feet together, stretch arms out in front, palms upright and facing out, and look ahead.

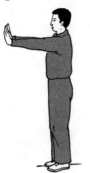

Breathe 10–20 times in this position. When breathing in, push palms forward with force and bend fingers backward. Relax arms when breathing out.

LEADING AN OX TO PULL GRAIN

Repeat preparation position. Step to right and turn body to right, bend right leg and keep left leg straight. Raise right fist high with elbow bent and keep left hand just behind back with fist clenched.

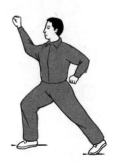

Breathe 5–10 times in this position. When breathing in, clench fists tightly and bend them in toward body; relax arms when breathing out. Repeat exercise, but to the left.

HAULING GRAIN ON THE BACK

Repeat preparation position. Place left hand on back, palm facing out, fingers reaching up as far as possible. Put right hand over shoulder and pull fingers of left hand.

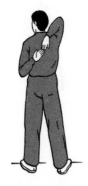

Breathe 5–10 times in this position. When breathing in, pull fingers; relax when breathing out. Change hands and repeat exercise.

Physical effects Strengthens muscles in chest, back and shoulders.

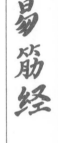

易
筋
经

UNLOADING GRAIN IN THE BASKET

Repeat preparation position.

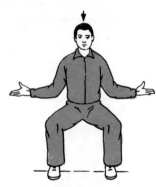

Step to left, bend knees to assume horse-riding position. Keep upper body straight, stretch arms out to side, palms up as though holding up a heavy object. Remain in this position for a moment and breathe in.

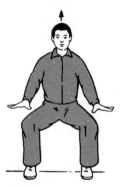

Turn palms over as though putting down a heavy object, breathe out and slowly get up until legs are straight and feet are together.
Repeat exercise many times.

Physical effects Strengthens muscles in legs, abdomen and also back.

PUTTING UP MATS AROUND GRAIN

Repeat preparation position. Stand straight with feet together. Clench left fist and hold at waist, reach out to left with right hand, fingers curled. Turn upper body to left, bend forward, twist round to right and straighten up. When twisting waist, move right hand in a circular motion as though putting up mats around grain.

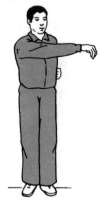

Repeat exercise 5–10 times in coordination with breathing. Breathe in when body is straight and left hand is close to waist; breathe out when bending body and stretching arm. Change hands and repeat exercise.

CATCHING GRAIN-EATING INSECTS

Repeat preparation position. Step to right and, with left leg straight, bend right knee. Bend down to right and, keeping head up, touch ground with both hands.

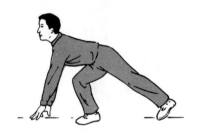

Breathe 10–20 times in this position. When breathing in, straighten arms and lift chest up;

when breathing out, bend arms and lower chest. Repeat exercise, but in opposite direction.

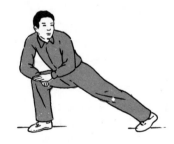

This movement is similar to a farmer searching for and catching grain-eating insects. It can also be done with hands resting on knee instead of touching ground.

Physical effects When done regularly, increases body strength and enhances equilibrium.

BENDING DOWN TO GATHER GRAIN

Repeat preparation position.

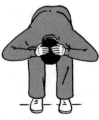

Hold back of head tightly with both hands and tap head with fingers for a few minutes. Bend body, put head between knees and breathe out; straighten body and breathe in. Repeat exercise 10–20 times.

Physical effects Helps to strengthen muscles in back, and tapping back of head with fingers is meant to help the memory.

BOWING TO SCOOP UP GRAIN

*Repeat preparation position.
Stand with feet apart, bend
forward, keep knees straight, arms
hanging, palms up; with head
raised try to touch ground with
backs of hands.*

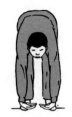

*Breathe out and lift heels when
bending down; breathe in and lower
heels when getting up.
Repeat exercise about 20 times.*

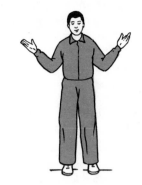

*Finally, spread arms to side and
bend and stretch arms seven times.*

THE THIRD SET

*This set is divided into 10 sections
and is done with clenched fists. The
10 movements need not be done in
rhythm with breathing since the
emphasis is on concentration, using
thoughts to direct motions. While
rigidity is to be avoided, the whole
body must be coordinated in support
of one particular movement and this
is the essence of all yijinjings.
They are not as simple as they look
since inner force must be utilized.
Each movement may be repeated up
to 50 times, depending on one's
physical condition and needs.*

THUMB LIFTING

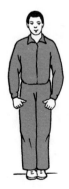

*Stand to attention. Place fists in
front of thighs, clench fingers and
point thumbs at each other. Use
inner force to lift thumbs while
tightening fingers and tensing whole
body as much as possible.
Relax and repeat exercise.*

THUMB HOLDING

*Stand with feet shoulder-width
apart, arms by side. Bend thumbs
and clench fingers over thumbs.*

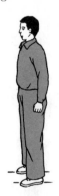

*In this position use inner force to
tighten fists while tensing whole
body as much as possible.*

ARMS FORWARD

*Stand with feet together, toes
pointing forward. Bend thumbs and
clench fingers over thumbs. Slowly
raise arms in front to shoulder level,
elbows slightly bent, fists facing
each other with a distance of 12 in
(30 cm) between them.*

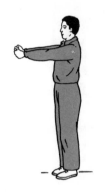

*In this position use inner force to
tighten fists while tensing whole
body. Relax and repeat exercise.*

ARMS UPWARD

*Stand with heels together but with
feet facing out. Bend thumbs and
clench fingers over thumbs.
Raise arms slowly, elbows slightly
bent, fists facing each other about
18 in (50 cm) apart.* ▶

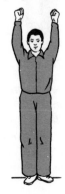

易筋经

In this position use inner force to tighten fists while heels are lifted and whole body is tensed up. Relax and lower heels.
Repeat exercise.

FISTS CLOSE TO EARS

Stand with feet shoulder-width apart, toes facing out. Bend thumbs, clench fingers over thumbs and raise arms to side, then bend forearms so that fists are close to ears.

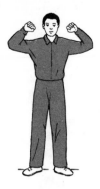

In this position use inner force to tighten fists while tensing whole body as much as possible.
Relax and repeat exercise.

TOE LIFTING

Stand with heels together but with toes facing out. Bend thumbs, clench fingers over thumbs and raise arms sideways up to shoulder level.

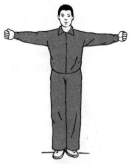

Lift toes off ground, press arms backward to cause upper body to lean back a little and, in this position, use inner force to tighten fists while whole body is tensed up. Relax, lower toes to ground and repeat exercise.

FISTS CLOSE TO NOSE

Stand with heels together but with toes facing out. Bend thumbs, clench fingers over thumbs and stretch arms to side, then bend forearms to bring fists close to nose, about 2 in (5 cm) apart, palms of fists facing out.

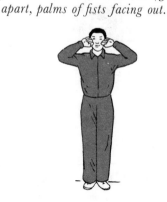

In this position use inner force to tighten fists while tensing whole body as much as possible.
Relax and repeat exercise.

FISTS UPRIGHT

Stand with heels together but with toes facing out. Bend thumbs, clench fingers over thumbs and stretch arms to side, then bend forearms and hold fists upright, palms facing out.

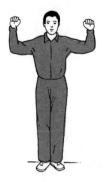

In this position, use inner force to tighten fists while tensing whole body as much as possible.
Relax and repeat exercise.

FISTS AT NAVEL

Stand with heels together but with toes facing out. Bend thumbs, clench fingers over thumbs and place fists by navel.

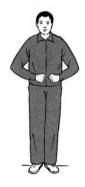

In this position use inner force to tighten fists while tensing whole body as much as possible.
Relax and repeat exercise.

FISTS BY CHEST

Stand with feet shoulder-width apart. Bend thumbs, clench fingers over thumbs and stretch arms to side, then bend forearms to bring fists to chest, palms down.

In this position use inner force to tighten fists while tensing whole body as much as possible.
Relax and repeat exercise.

When you have completed the 10 movements, breathe deeply three to five times.

电子工人操

COFFEE BREAK EXERCISES

In China, factory and office workers take a break for exercises in much the same way as we in the West take coffee breaks. The exercises shown here are popular throughout China, where they are called production exercises. They are simple, easy to learn and suitable for both young and old. Each should be done in precise motion and it is helpful to count the steps in rhythm as you go along.

HEAD

THE FIRST SET

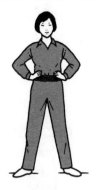 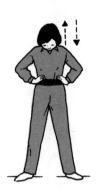 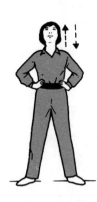 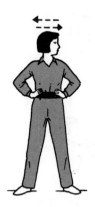 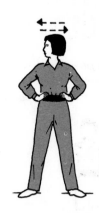

Preparation *Stand straight, feet apart, hands at waist.*
1–2 *Drop head forward and bring it back twice.*

3–4 *Stretch head back and bring it straight back again twice.*
5–6 *Turn head to left and to front again twice.*

7–8 *Turn head to right and to front again twice.*

THE SECOND SET

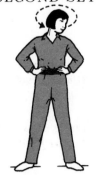 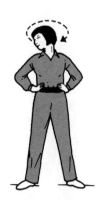

1–4 *Close eyes and rotate head to left four times.*

5–8 *Close eyes and rotate head to right four times.*
Repeat exercise four times.

Points to remember
● *When rotating head, count steps slowly.*

Physical effects Relieves fatigue in neck muscles and is therefore suitable for those who work with their heads bent.

ARMS

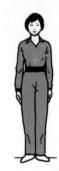

電
子
工
人
操

THE FIRST SET

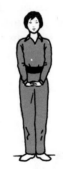 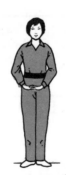 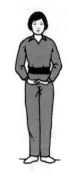

Preparation *Stand to attention.*
1 Interlock fingers, stretch arms and push down with palms open.

2 Bend elbows and lift hands slightly.

3–4 Repeat steps 1–2.

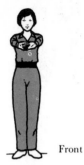 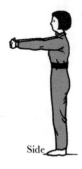 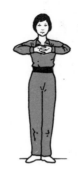 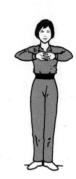

Front   Side

5 With fingers still interlocked and elbows bent, bring hands to chest. Stretch arms straight out with backs of hands facing body.

6 Bend elbows and bring hands back to chest.

7 Stretch arms out again.
8 Repeat step 6.

THE SECOND SET

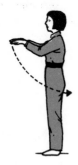 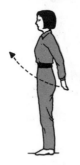

1 Relax elbows and throw arms back.

2 Swing arms forward.
3–8 Repeat steps 1–2 three times. Repeat exercise four times.

Points to remember
● *When interlocking fingers, stretch arms down and out as far as possible.*
● *When swinging arms backward and forward, relax fingers, wrists and arms.*

Physical effects Relieves stiffness in arms, wrists and fingers and is therefore especially effective for those who do delicate work with fingers.

CHEST

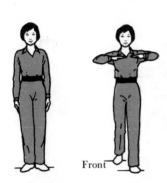
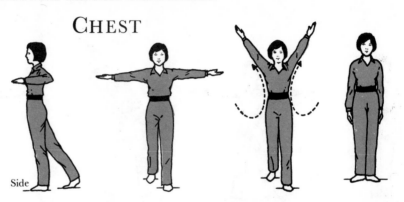

电子工人操

Preparation *Stand to attention.*
1 *Step forward with left leg and shift weight to left foot. Lift right heel off ground and bring hands up to chest pointing at each other, palms down.*
2 *Stretch arms out to side with palms up.*

3 *Keeping head up and chest out, move arms down and up in curves.*
4 *Return to preparation position.*
5–8 *Repeat steps 1–4, but with right foot forward.*
Repeat exercise four times.

Points to remember
● *Push chest out as far as possible.*

● *When lifting arms up, keep them straight.*

Physical effects Relaxes chest muscles, straightens vertebral column and regulates breathing. It also eliminates fatigue and is especially beneficial for those who have to bend a lot.

LEGS

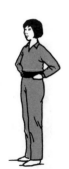
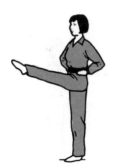
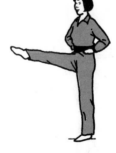

Preparation *Stand straight, hands at waist.*

1 *Throw left leg up as high as possible.*
2 *Lower left leg.*

3 *Throw right leg up as high as possible.*
4 *Lower right leg.*

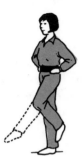
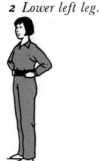
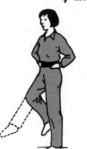

5 *Lift left leg with knee bent and kick forward.*
6 *Lower left leg.*
7 *Lift right leg with knee bent and kick forward.*
8 *Lower right leg.*

Repeat exercise four times and then stand to attention, arms by side.

Points to remember
● *When kicking keep toes pointed and leg straight.*

Physical effects Increases blood circulation in lower limbs and helps relieve fatigue of workers who spend most of their day sitting down.

SIDES

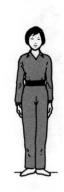
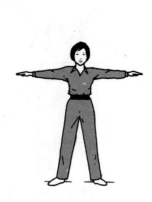
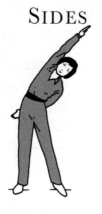
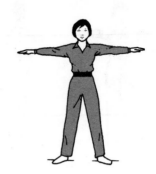
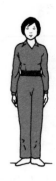

Preparation *Stand to attention.*
1 Step to left and stretch arms out to side, palms down.
2 Stretch right arm high above head, bend body to left. Put left arm down behind back and lift left foot up so that only toes are touching ground.

3 Repeat step 1.
4 Return to preparation position.
5–8 Repeat steps 1–4, but in opposite direction.

Points to remember
● *When bending to side keep head and raised arm straight.*

Physical effects Strengthens waist muscles and increases blood circulation. Eliminates fatigue of workers who spend most of their day sitting down.

BODY TWISTING

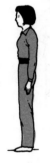
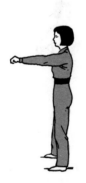
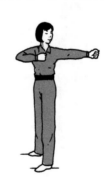
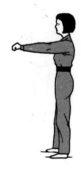
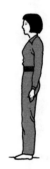

Preparation *Stand to attention.*
1 Stretch arms out in front, clench fists, palms down. At same time step to left.
2 Twist body to left together with left arm, palm facing forward. At same time bend right arm, palm facing chest.

3 Repeat step 1.
4 Return to preparation position.
5–8 Repeat steps 1–4, but in opposite direction.

Points to remember
● *When twisting body, keep legs straight and feet still.*

Physical effects Strengthens muscles in abdomen and back. Helps relieve fatigue of workers who spend most of their day sitting down.

THE WHOLE BODY

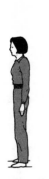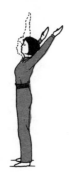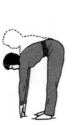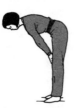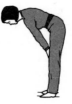

Preparation *Stand to attention.*
1 Raise arms straight up, palms facing out. Keeping head high and chest out, bend upper body back and return to upright position.
2 Keeping arms straight, bend upper body back again.
3 With straight knees, bend forward and touch ground.

4 Raise upper body slightly and bend down again to touch ground.
5 Keeping knees together and feet on ground, place hands on knees and squat.
6 Straighten legs, keep body bent and touch knees.
7–8 Repeat steps 5–6.

Repeat exercise four times and return to preparation position.

Points to remember
● *When bending back, keep arms and legs straight.*

Physical effects Increases circulation and relaxes body.

LIMBERING UP

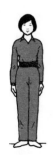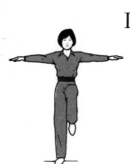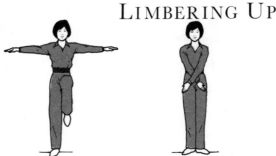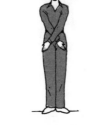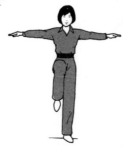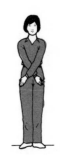

Preparation *Stand to attention.*
1 Stretch arms out to side, palms down, and lift left knee.

2 Return to preparation position and cross arms in front of body.

3 Stretch arms out to side, palms down, and lift right knee.
4 Repeat step 2.

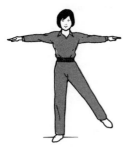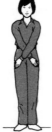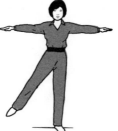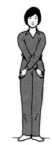
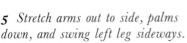

5 Stretch arms out to side, palms down, and swing left leg sideways.
6 Repeat step 2.
7 Stretch arms out to side, palms down, and swing right leg sideways.
8 Repeat step 2.
Repeat exercise twice and return to preparation position.

Points to remember
● *All limbs must be completely relaxed.*
● *March on spot twice, before and after exercise, each time to a count of eight.*

Physical effects Relaxes muscles of whole body, regulates breathing, and therefore enables workers to return to work with renewed energy.

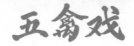

ANIMAL PLAY

A variety of forms of the five animal play exercises has evolved through the ages. The three sets described here are the most popular among workers. The following rules, however, must be adhered to so that the fullest possible benefit is derived from the exercises. Relax the whole body and do the exercises regularly and concentrate on the lower abdomen. Breathing must be natural and plenty of fresh air is necessary. Since these movements originated from the movements of animals it is important to imitate the motions and manners of these animals as you are exercising. Do not exercise within one hour of eating.

There are several physical effects: tiger play strengthens the body; deer play relaxes muscles; monkey play increases nimbleness of limbs; bear play is good for internal organs; and crane play is good for lungs and helps circulation.

SIMPLIFIED EXERCISES

These exercises are suitable for beginners, the elderly and the infirm.

THE TIGER IMAGE

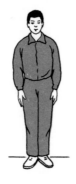

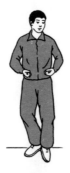

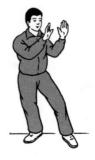

Preparation *Stand to attention, but do not attempt to push chest out. Relax whole body in this position for a few moments.*
1 Bend knees slowly and lower body, shifting weight to right leg.

Lift left heel to touch right ankle bone and at same time bring fists to waist, palms up, eyes looking toward left.
2 Step forward to left, follow with right foot until distance between two

heels is about 12 in (30 cm) and keep weight on right leg. At same time move fists to chest level and push forward with open palms, eyes looking at left forefinger.

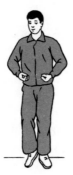

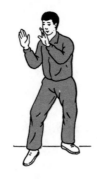

3 Move left foot half a step forward and touch left ankle bone with right heel, knees slightly bent in a squatting position. At same

time bring fists to waist, palms up, eyes looking toward right.
4 Repeat step 2, but in opposite direction.

Repeat exercise to left and right many times in a calm and composed manner, similar to that of a confident tiger preparing for battle.

THE BEAR IMAGE

THE MONKEY IMAGE

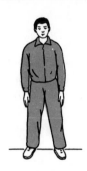

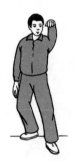

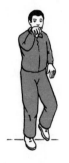

Preparation *Stand naturally with feet shoulder-width apart and arms by side. Breathe deeply three to five times.*

Preparation *Stand to attention and relax body in this position for a few moments.*

1 Bend knees slowly and step forward with left foot; at same time move left hand up along chest to shoulder level, thrust it forward as though grabbing an object and, with wrist bent, form claw with hand.

2 Step forward with right foot and follow with left foot, its heel lifted off ground; at same time move right hand up along chest to shoulder level, thrust it forward as though grabbing an object and, with wrist bent, form claw with hand. Draw left hand back, elbow bent.

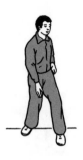

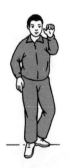

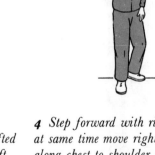

1 Bend right knee and sway right shoulder forward and down, arm hanging; at same time pull left shoulder back and lift left arm slightly.

3 Step back with left foot and follow with right foot, its heel lifted off ground; at same time move left hand up along chest to shoulder level, thrust it forward as though grabbing an object and, with wrist bent, form claw with hand. Draw right hand back, elbow bent.

4 Step forward with right foot and at same time move right hand up along chest to shoulder level, thrust it forward as though grabbing an object and, with wrist bent, form hand into claw. Draw left hand back, elbow bent.

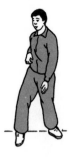

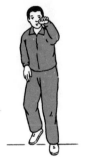

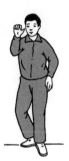

2 Repeat step 1, but in opposite direction.
Repeat exercise many times.

5–6 Repeat steps 2–3, but in opposite direction.

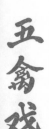

THE DEER IMAGE

Preparation *Stand to attention and relax body in this position for a few moments.*

1 *Bend right leg and stretch left leg forward with knee slightly bent. Put weight on right leg.*

2 *Stretch left arm forward, elbow slightly bent and place right hand in position where its palm faces left elbow.*

3 *Rotate arms counter-clockwise, making sure that circle drawn by left hand is larger and that rotation of arms is brought about by circular*

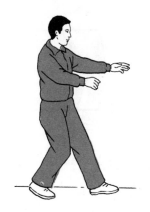

motion of hips and waist and not by movement of shoulder joints. Repeat movement a few times.

4–6 *Repeat steps 1–3, but put right leg and arm forward, hold left hand in position where palm faces right elbow and rotate arms clockwise.*

Repeat exercise to left and right many times.

Physical effects Especially good for kidneys, circulation of lower body and helps to strengthen leg muscles.

THE CRANE IMAGE

Preparation *Stand naturally and relax for a few moments.*

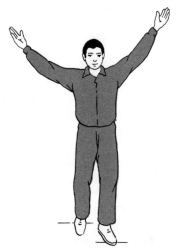

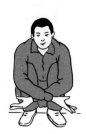

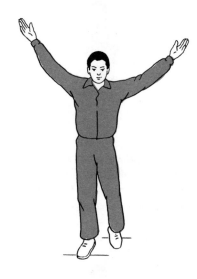

1 *Step forward with left foot, take half a step forward with right foot, heel off ground; at same time raise hands in front, spread them out to side and breathe in.*

2 *Take half a step forward with right foot, lower arms, squat, hug knees and breathe out.*

3 *Get up, step forward with right foot, take half a step forward with left foot, heel off ground; at same time raise hands in front, spread them out to sides and breathe in.*

4 *Repeat step 2, but move left foot forward.*

Physical effects Strengthens heart, lungs, kidneys and waist.

20 VARIATIONS

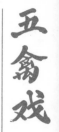

Try and do at least 100 of the steps explained below, alternating movements to left and right. Move slowly and keep your posture low.

These exercises should be done in a continuous flow. The arrows explain the action leading to the position in the following figure and should always be followed carefully.

LIMBERING UP TO GET READY

FIRST MOVEMENT

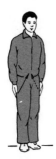 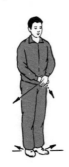 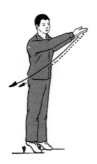 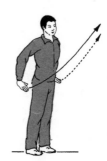 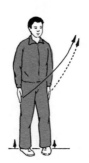

Preparation *Stand to attention.*
1 Place hands against abdomen and relax whole body.
2–3 Move feet sideways until legs are shoulder-width apart. With fingers together and arms by side, turn feet slightly in.
4–5 Swing arms backward and forward 30 times; when swinging arms forward, turn palms up, lift heels and breathe in; when swinging arms backward, keep head and chest out and press hands down with palms turned over, lower heels and breathe out.

SECOND MOVEMENT
Preparation *Stand with feet shoulder-width apart, feet turned slightly in and knees bent.*
1 Swing left arm forward, right arm back, palms up, and breathe in.
2 Swing right arm forward, left arm back, palms up, and breathe out. Do exercise 30 times and then repeat with right arm swung up first.

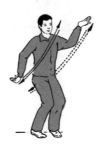

THIRD MOVEMENT
Preparation *Stand with feet shoulder-width apart, feet turned slightly in and knees out.*

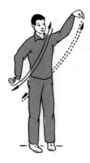 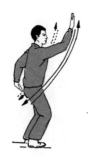

1 Bend wrists, swing left arm up, palm down, right arm back, palm up, and breathe in.

2 Unbend wrists, bend knees and repeat movement with alternate arms. Do exercise 30 times and then repeat with right arm swung up first.

五禽戏

CONCLUSION

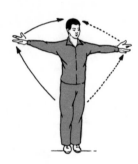

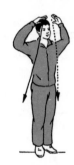

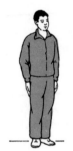

This exercise should be done after each movement.
1 *Stand naturally, stretch arms out to side, turn palms up.*

2 *Lift heels, bring arms above head, bring hands down and breathe out deeply.*

3 *Lower heels and return to standing naturally.*

THE FIRST FIVE VARIATIONS

THE TIGER

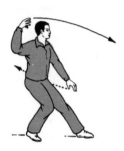

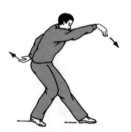

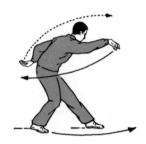

Preparation *Stand naturally.*
1 *Step forward with left foot, bend right knee; thrust right arm up and forward with hand shaped like a*

tiger's claw, palm down, and throw left arm behind back, palm up.
2 *Stretch arms a few times in this position.*

3 *Push right arm down, left arm up, step forward with right foot and repeat exercise on opposite side.*

THE DEER

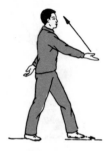

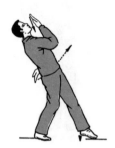

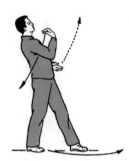

Preparation *Stand naturally.*
1 *Step forward with left foot and lean back.*

2 *Lift right hand toward face, keeping eyes on palm, hold left hand behind back, palm up, and, keeping chest high, stretch neck.*

3 *Bring right arm down, left arm up, right foot forward and repeat exercise on opposite side.*

THE MONKEY

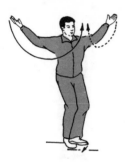 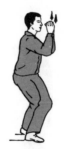 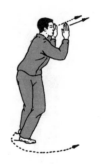

Preparation *Stand naturally.*
1 Cross left leg over right leg, toes pointing to left; stretch arms out as far as possible, clench fists and bring them together at eye level.
2 Turn head to left and squat; at same time unclench fists, keep finger tips level with forehead and blink eyes at least three times.
3 Cross right leg over left leg and repeat exercise on opposite side.

THE BEAR

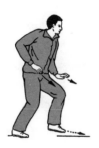 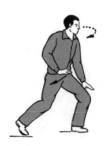 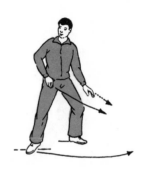

Preparation *Stand naturally.*
1 Step forward with left foot and bend both knees. Keep arms close to body and stretch left hand forward, palm down, and keep right hand at waist, palm down.
2 With right arm close to body, turn to right.
3 Move right foot forward, stretch right hand forward as far as possible, push left arm down and repeat exercise on opposite side.

THE CRANE

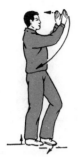 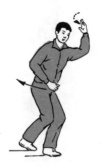 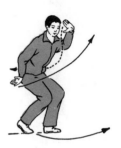

Preparation *Stand naturally.*
1 Cross left leg over right leg and bend knees slightly. Raise and cross arms, palms facing out.
2 Turn left palm in and put right hand behind back, palm up.
3 Squat and turn body to right. Cross right leg over left leg, move right arm up and left arm down and repeat exercise on opposite side.

THE SECOND FIVE VARIATIONS

THE TIGER

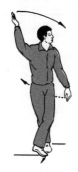
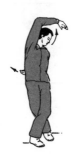
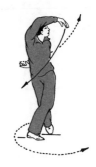

Preparation *Stand naturally.*
1 Cross left leg over right leg, raise right hand and move it in a curve to left, palm down; at same time move left hand behind back, palm up.

2 Twist body to left and look at right heel.
3 Lift head and gaze ahead for a moment in imitation of a tiger searching for prey. Move right hand

down, left arm up, cross right leg over left leg and repeat exercise on opposite side.

THE DEER

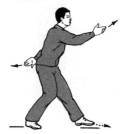
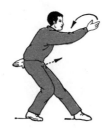
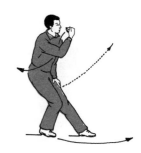

Preparation *Stand naturally.*
1 Step forward with left foot, bend right knee; at same time reach out with right hand, palm facing left, thumb level with nose, and move left

hand behind back, palm facing right, thumb down.
2 Lower body; bring left hand forward and bend right arm into body at chest level.

3 Bring right arm behind back, left arm up, right foot forward and repeat exercise on opposite side.

THE MONKEY

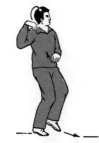
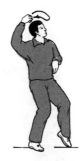
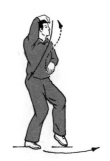

Preparation *Stand naturally.*
1 Bend knees slightly, lift left heel off ground and step forward; at same time hold left arm close to chest, fingers hanging, and lift right arm with fingers and wrist bent so

that they are level with shoulder.
2 Lift right arm with elbow bent above head and move it in a circular motion from back of head to front, with thumb, forefinger and middle finger curled like those of a monkey

when picking fruit off trees.
3 Bring right arm down and left arm up and repeat exercise on opposite side.

THE BEAR

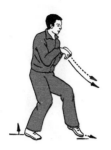 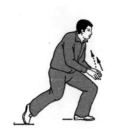 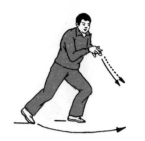

Preparation *Stand naturally.*
1 Step forward with left foot, heel off ground, knee bent and abdomen contracted.

2 At same time bend right knee slightly, lift heel off ground and stretch hands down, with left foot firmly on ground.

3 Bring hands down, step forward with right foot and repeat exercise on opposite side.

THE CRANE

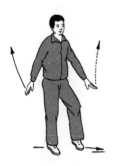 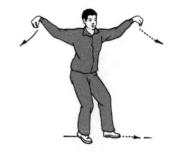 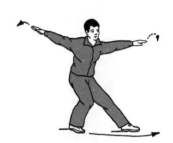

Preparation *Stand naturally.*
1 Step forward gently with left foot, bend right knee slightly and hold arms out to side.

2 Raise arms with wrists bent and fingers hanging.
3 Lower body slightly, straighten left leg and stretch arms. Bring

right foot forward, lower arms and repeat exercise on opposite side.

THE THIRD FIVE VARIATIONS

THE TIGER

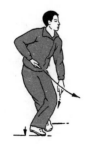 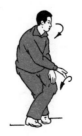 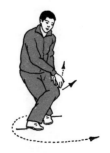

Preparation *Stand naturally.*
1 Cross left leg over right leg and squat; at same time lower left hand, bend right elbow and thrust right

hand down as far as possible.
2 Put left hand on left knee and turn right hand over, palm down, and turn head to right.

3 Cross right leg over left leg, lower right hand, bend left elbow, thrust left hand down and repeat exercise on opposite side.

五禽戲

THE DEER

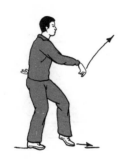
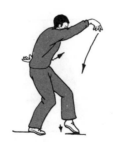
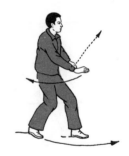

Preparation *Stand naturally.*
1 Step forward with left leg, heel off ground, and lean forward; at same time bend right knee slightly and raise right arm with wrist bent

and fingers hanging. Keep left arm behind back with fingers pointing up.
2 Lower right arm and bring left arm forward.

3 Bring right arm behind back, raise left arm and repeat exercise on opposite side.

THE MONKEY

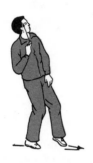
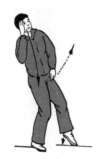
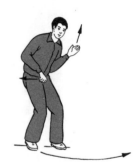

Preparation *Stand naturally.*
1 Step forward with left leg, heel off ground, heel twisted outward, and lean back slightly.

2 At same time, keeping left arm close to body, fingers hanging, lift right hand and rest all five fingers on forehead above right eyebrow;

look up toward left.
3 Move left arm up, lower right arm as far as possible and repeat exercise on opposite side.

THE BEAR

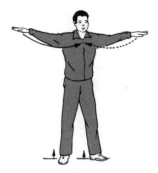
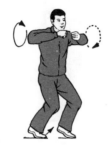
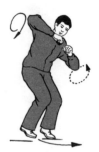

Preparation *Stand naturally.*
1 Bend knees, lift heels off ground, stretch arms out to side, palms down.

2 Bend elbows, clench fists and hold them at chest level under chin.
3 Step to left and make circular

movements with both elbows.
4 Step to right and make circular movements with elbows.

THE CRANE

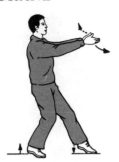 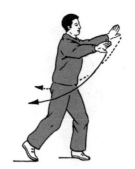 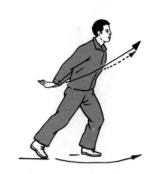

Preparation *Stand naturally.*
1 Step forward with left leg, bend right knee slightly and throw arms forward, palms facing each other.
2 Turn palms outward, bring arms behind back in a curve, with palms facing up.
3 Push chest forward, pull shoulders back and, with right heel lifted off ground, put weight on left foot.
4 Push arms forward, step forward with right foot and repeat exercise on opposite side.

THE FOURTH FIVE VARIATIONS

THE TIGER

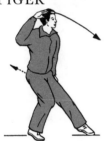 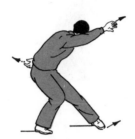 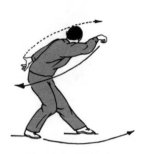

Preparation *Stand naturally.*
1 Step forward with left foot, lift heel off ground and turn toes in; at same time bend right knee, form hands into claws and bring right hand level with head.
2 Thrust right arm forward, palm facing out, twist body to left and throw left arm behind back, palm up. When twisting body, open eyes and mouth wide and stick out tongue in imitation of face of a fierce tiger.
3 Bring right arm behind back, left arm level with head, right foot forward and repeat movement on opposite side.

THE DEER

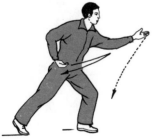 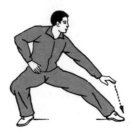 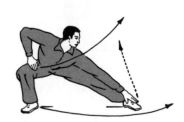

Preparation *Stand naturally.*
1 Step forward with left foot, thrust hands forward, palms up; draw right arm back and press left hand down as far as possible.
2 At same time turn right foot and right knee to right and, with left leg straight, lower body. Hold right hand just above knee and tap left foot with left hand three times.
3 Bring arms up and repeat exercise on opposite side.

五禽戲

THE MONKEY

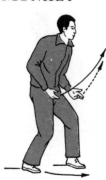

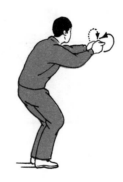

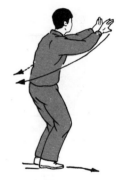

Preparation *Stand naturally.*
1–2 *Step to left, bring feet together and bend knees; at same time move*

arms up in a curve, palms up. Close fingers in imitation of a monkey picking fruits.

3 *With palms open, swing arms back in a curve.*

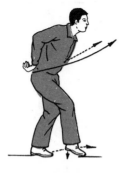

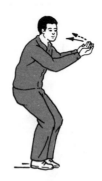

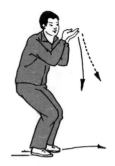

4–6 *Step to right, bring feet together and bend knees; at same time move arms up in a curve, palms*

up and open, in imitation of a monkey offering fruits.

THE BEAR

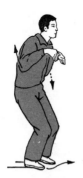

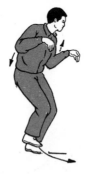

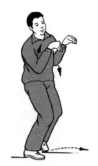

Preparation *Stand naturally.*
1 *Raise forearms with wrists bent and fingers hanging, hold upper*

arms close to body and bend knees.
2 *Step to left, lift right foot slightly off ground, bend upper body*

and swing head to left.
3 *Step to right and repeat exercise on opposite side.*

THE CRANE

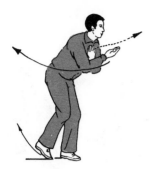 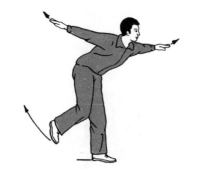 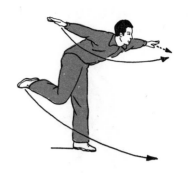

Preparation *Stand naturally.*
1 Step forward with left leg, bend right knee and lift heel off ground. At same time cross arms in front of chest and lean forward.

2 Stretch arms to side, palms down; at same time bend right knee further so that sole of foot is facing up. Stretch neck, push head forward and gently roll eyes.

3 Cross arms again, bring right foot forward and repeat exercise on opposite side.

CONCLUSION

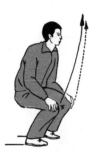 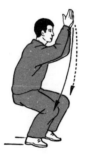 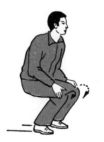

Preparation *Stand naturally and relax, as the purpose of this movement is to relieve the fatigue caused by the previous exercises.*

1 Look straight ahead and bend knees to assume a horse-riding position. Slap buttocks and thighs.
2 Raise hands and clap once.

3 Rest hands on knees.
4 Shake shoulders and knees.

ADVANCED EXERCISES

Preparation *Stand naturally with feet shoulder-width apart and parallel to each other; keep arms hanging at side.*

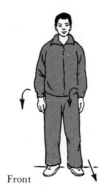

Front

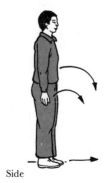

Side

TIGER PLAY

五禽戲

PRYING ABOUT TO THE RIGHT

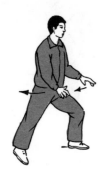
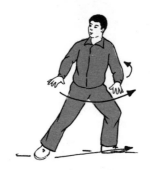

1 Step forward with left foot and, keeping right knee straight, bend left knee; at same time lean forward, bend elbows and hold hands above left thigh, fingers spread out and pointing down like tigers' claws.

2 Turn slowly as far as you can to right, following movement with eyes that are alert and searching like those of a hungry tiger.

3 Turn back slowly, eyes following movement.

PRYING ABOUT TO THE LEFT

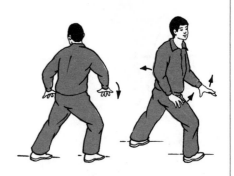

Repeat steps 1–3 of Prying about to the right, but in opposite direction. Pry to left and right at least twice.

Points to remember

● *Move as though you are a fierce and hungry tiger with a light and nimble body.*

● *Move neck and body together, breathe normally and keep eyes alert.*

CLAWING TO THE LEFT

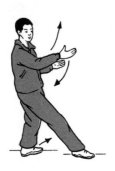
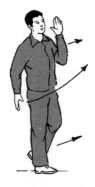
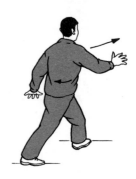

1 Following lines of step 3 of Prying about to the left, raise arms slowly, left palm facing right wrist and lean back so that weight is on left leg.

2 Lean forward and shift weight to right leg; at same time lift left foot, raise left hand to eye level and drop right arm to side.

3 Stamp right foot, step forward with left foot and, keeping right leg straight, bend left leg. Form hands into claws and thrust left hand down and right arm forward and move body 45 degrees to left.

CLAWING TO THE RIGHT

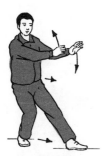 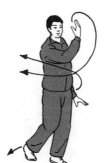 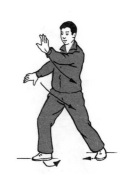

Repeat steps 1–3 of Clawing to the left, but in opposite direction.

MAULING TO THE LEFT

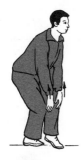 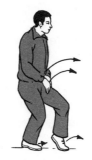 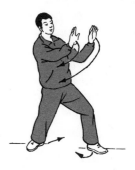

1 *Following lines of step 3 of Clawing to the right, pivot on ball of right foot, its heel twisted out 45 degrees, and turn 90 degrees to left; at same time lift left foot and place*

its toes in front of right foot; keep chest in, abdomen contracted and place hands on left knee.
2 *Straighten body slowly and lift hands up.*

3 *Stamp right foot and step forward with left foot; keeping right leg straight, bend left leg and at same time thrust hands forward.*

MAULING TO THE RIGHT

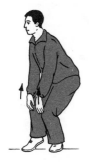 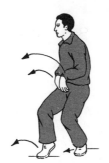 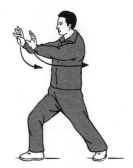

Repeat steps 1–3 of Mauling to the left, but in opposite direction.

Points to remember
● *When thrusting hands forward, be spry and swift and spread fingers out like tigers' claws.*
● *When stamping foot and moving forward, roar like a tiger.*

GRAPPLING – FRONT ATTACK

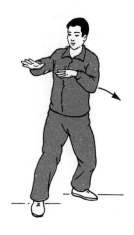

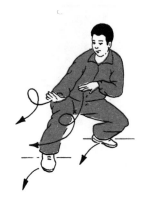

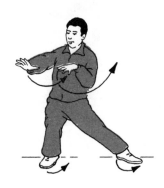

1 Following lines of step 3 of Mauling to the right, pivot on ball of right foot, heel turned out 45 degrees, step back with left foot and put weight on left leg; at same time stretch right hand forward and bring left hand back to chest, palms down, fingers spread out.

2 Sway body forward and backward and, following lines of arrows, draw circles. When swaying forward, bend right knee and keep left leg straight. When swaying backward, bend left knee and keep right leg straight, shifting weight backward and forward.

3 Repeat step 2 but after backward sway, skip forward first with left foot then with right and at same time form hands into claws and thrust them forward as though attacking.

GRAPPLING – REAR ATTACK

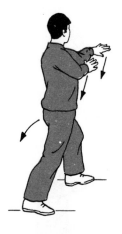

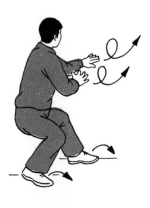

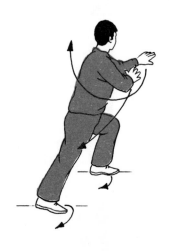

1 Pivot on balls of both feet, turn 180 degrees to left and place weight on right leg; at same time stretch left hand forward and bring right hand to chest, fingers spread out.

2 Repeat step 2 of Front attack, but when swaying forward bend left knee and keep right leg straight and when swaying backward bend right knee and keep right leg straight.

3 Repeat step 3 of Front attack, but skip first with right foot then with left and attack with fingers.

Points to remember
● *Concentrate and imagine that you are grappling with an enemy.*
● *Coordinate movements of body and legs.*
● *Attack with force, with fingers spread out like spikes.*

TURNING TO THE RIGHT

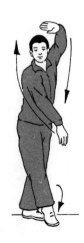

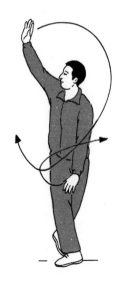

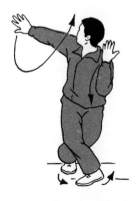

1 Following lines of step 3 of Grappling – rear attack, shift weight to right foot. Turn left foot about 140 degrees inward and keep both knees straight. Shift weight to left foot and take half a step back with right foot, heel off ground. At same time twist body to right, drop right hand in front of abdomen and lift left hand above forehead, palm facing out, and keep eyes firmly on back of hand.

2 Turn upper body slowly 90 degrees to right; at same time lift right hand up and bring left hand down toward right in a curve.

3 Bring right hand toward chest, palm down and left hand toward abdomen as though you are holding a ball; at same time squat, stretch right hand out and bend left elbow to bring left hand up to shoulder level; keep eyes on right hand.

TURNING TO THE LEFT

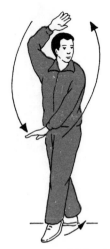

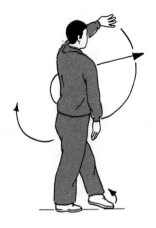

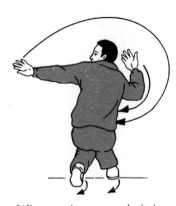

Repeat steps 1–3 of Turning to the right, but in opposite direction.

Points to remember
● *When turning, coordinate movement of limbs and relax muscles.*

● *When moving arms, do it in rhythm and at a wide angle.*

DEER PLAY

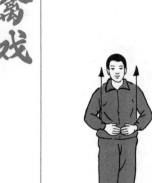

LOOKING FROM ABOVE TO THE LEFT

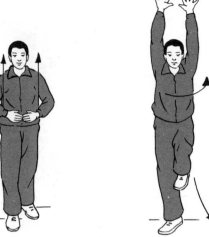

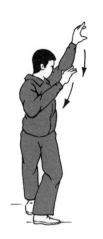

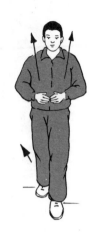

1 Following lines of step 3 of Turning to the left, stand up and make a full backward turn with weight on left foot; move right foot slightly forward and place both hands firmly against abdomen.

2 Raise arms high, fingers spread out, palms facing out; at same time, shift weight to right foot and lift left knee high.
3 Stamp left foot in front of right

foot and twist body to left, keeping eyes on left rear.
4 Turn body back and place hands against abdomen, left foot in front of right foot.

LOOKING FROM ABOVE TO THE RIGHT

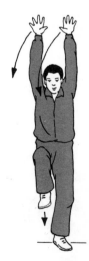

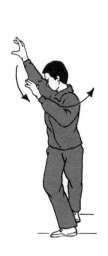

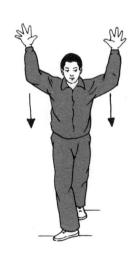

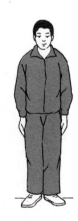

Repeat steps 2–4 of Looking from above to the left, but in opposite direction and assume a standing to attention position.

Points to remember
● *When raising arms, spread fingers out like deers' antlers.*
● *When standing on one leg, keep body steady.*
● *When lifting knee, thigh should be parallel to ground. Keep head high and look comfortable.*

BUTTING TO THE LEFT

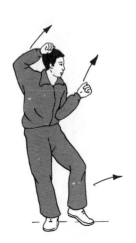 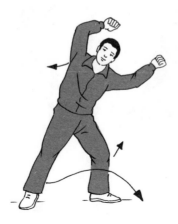 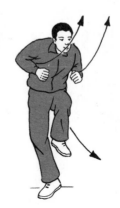 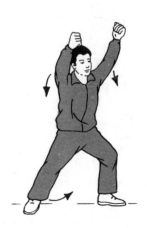

1 Put weight on right leg and lift left heel off ground; hold right fist by head and left fist low, with elbow touching abdomen; keep eyes on left fist.

2 Step forward to left and thrust head and fists toward left.
3 Bend elbows and draw arms back to waist; leap with right foot

forward to left; lean forward and lift left knee.
4 Stamp left foot hard, step to left and thrust fists up.

BUTTING TO THE RIGHT

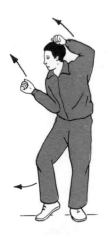 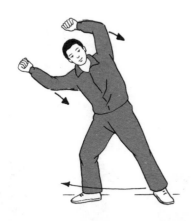 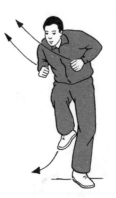 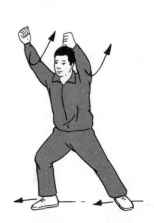

Repeat steps *1–4* of Butting to the left, but in opposite direction.

Points to remember
● When butting sideways, keep one elbow close to chest and raise the other.
● When stepping forward and thrusting fists up, use force and stretch upper body.
● All movements must be light and swift in imitation of the agility and nimbleness of a deer.

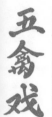

CIRCLE TWISTING TO THE LEFT

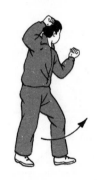 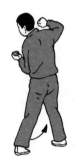 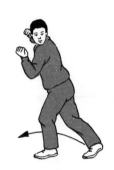 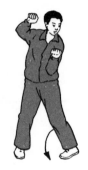 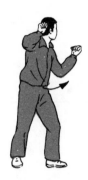

1 *Following lines of step 4 of Butting to the right, turn body to left, with right heel twisted out, and* *put weight on right foot. Bend left arm at waist, right arm by head and stamp left foot.*

2–5 *Lean to left and walk in a circle counter-clockwise in four steps, starting with right foot.*

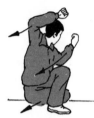 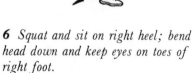 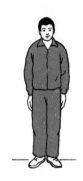

6 *Squat and sit on right heel; bend head down and keep eyes on toes of right foot.*

7 *Stand to attention.*

Points to remember
● *When turning circle, make each step about 18 in (45 cm) long; bend knees slightly and twist toes toward body with each step.*
● *When leaning in, make sure that inner fist is low, with elbow close to chest, and outer fist is high, with elbow stretched out.*
● *Eyes should follow movement of body, which should be relaxed and natural throughout exercise.*

CIRCLE TWISTING TO THE RIGHT

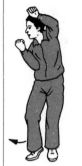 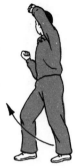 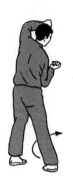 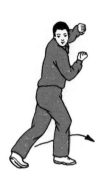 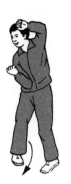 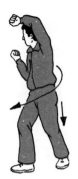 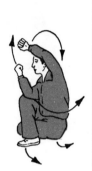

Repeat steps 1–7 of Circle twisting to the left, but in opposite direction.

BEAR PLAY

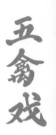

SWAYING

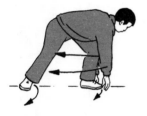
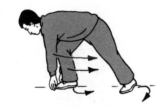

1 *Following lines of step 7 of Circle twisting to the right, turn to left, placing weight on left foot. Lift right heel off ground, bend down to touch left heel with left hand and toes with right hand.*

2 *Sway body to right and take a big step with right foot; lift left heel off ground, bend over and touch right heel with right hand and toes with left hand.*
3–4 *Repeat steps 1–2.*

Points to remember
● *When swaying, be slow and steady.*
● *Arms should be relaxed and hanging and should swing with shoulders; eyes should follow hands.*

PUSHING LEFT

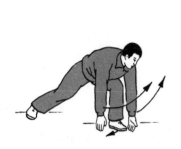
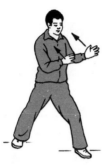
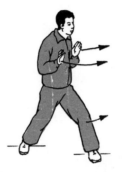

1–2 *Following lines of step 2 of Swaying, sway to left and get up. Place weight on left foot and bring hands up to waist level, palms facing each other.*

3 *Move upper body back, shift weight to right leg and draw arms back to chest, fingers pointing up and palms facing forward.*

4 *Push forward hard with hands, follow with body and shift weight to left leg.*
5–6 *Repeat steps 3–4.*

PUSHING RIGHT

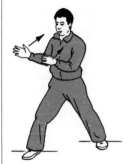
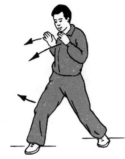
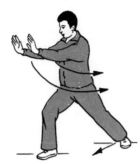

Repeat steps 2–4 of Pushing left, but in opposite direction and assume a natural standing position.

Points to remember
● *Make sure that movement of arms and legs is coordinated and in rhythm.*
● *When shifting weight back and forth, be natural and breathe deeply, with shoulders dropped and keep elbows as low as possible.*

五禽戲

CLIMBING

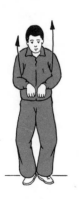 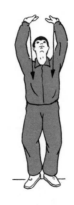 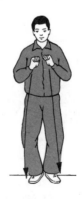 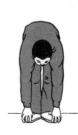 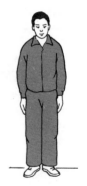

1 Hold hands at waist level as though holding a bar.
2 Stretch hands up, eyes following.
3 Lower hands slowly to chest as though pulling up on a single bar.

4 Bend forward and pull at toes.
5 Straighten body slowly and stand to attention.
Repeat exercise two or more times.

Points to remember
● *When pulling up and bending down to pull at toes, keep knees straight and legs stretched.*
● *Concentrate throughout exercise and breathe normally.*

MONKEY PLAY

LEAPING TO THE LEFT

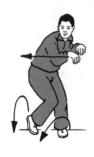 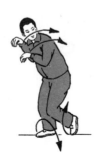 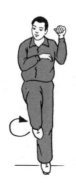 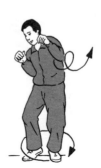 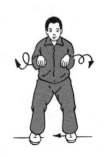

1 Hooking wrists and fingers like claws of a monkey, bring left hand to left shoulder and right hand to left side of chest; at same time bend knees, lift right heel off ground, placing weight on left foot, eyes leering to right.

2 Leap to right on right foot and draw right hand to right ear and left hand to right side of chest; shift weight to right foot with left heel off ground, eyes leering to left.
3 Leap to left and repeat step 1.
4 Lift right foot and draw a small circle clockwise.

5 Lower right foot and touch ground with toes.
6 Pivot on ball of right foot and make full circle turn quickly.
7 Place weight on both feet with knees bent, keep elbows close to chest with hands hooked and shake upper body a couple of times.

LEAPING TO THE RIGHT
Repeat steps 1–7 of Leaping to the left, but in opposite direction.

Points to remember
● *With hands hooked, elbows lifted and knees bent, you automatically assume the posture of a monkey.*
● *All movements including leaping and turning must be swift.*

PICKING AND OFFERING FRUITS TO THE RIGHT

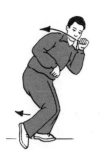 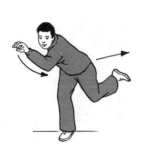 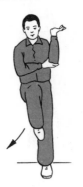 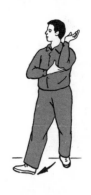 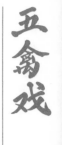

1 Bring left hand close to left ear and right hand to left side of chest; lift right leg and put weight on left leg, eyes leering to right.
2 Leap to right, landing on right foot and lean forward; at same time

reach out with left hand in imitation of a monkey picking fruit. Stretch left leg back.
3 Straighten body and leap to left, landing on left foot; at same time lift right knee and draw right hand

to hold left elbow so that left forearm is upright, palm facing up in imitation of a monkey presenting fruit.
4 Drop right foot to ground and point toes to right.

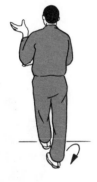 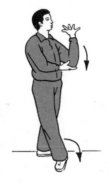

5 Move left foot a step forward in front of right foot and turn to right and then back.
6 Step forward with right foot, twist toes as much as you can to

right and continue to turn to right.
7 Step forward with left foot and continue to turn.
8 Bring feet together, drop hands and return to a standing position.

Points to remember
● *Movements must be quick.*
● *When leaping to pick fruit, lean forward and balance body with back leg stretched out.*

PICKING AND OFFERING FRUITS TO THE LEFT

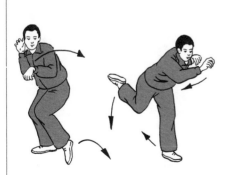 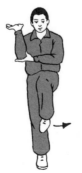 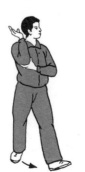 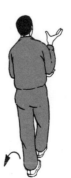 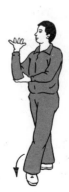 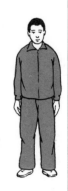

Repeat steps 1–8 of Picking and offering fruits to the right, but in opposite direction.

MONKEY BREATHING

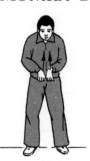 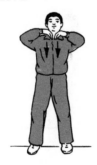 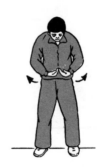

1 Stand with feet apart, hold hands together in front of abdomen and look at backs of hands.
2 Lift hands slowly and breathe in, keeping eyes on hands. As hands gradually reach level of throat your lungs should be full of air.
3 Turn hands over, pull downward and breathe out. At same time bend forward slowly. As you breathe out say ho . . . hu . . . si . . . shoo . . . shee . . . tsui. . . .

Points to remember
● *Relax and be natural.*
● *Breathing must be long, slow and even.*
● *When breathing out, say the given six words. Legend has it that such a method of breathing out may help prevent diseases of the internal organs.*

MONKEY MASSAGE

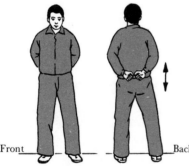 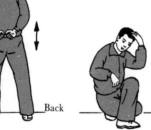 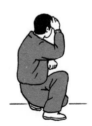 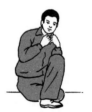 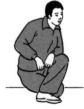

Front   Back

1 To massage waist clench fists loosely, rub waist and lower back 30 times with knuckles, then pound same area 30 times and squat.

2 Step forward to right with left foot and sit on right foot with right knee on ground. Peep around and scratch yourself all over.

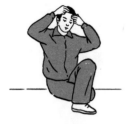

3 Use forefingers and middle fingers to massage the following points: back of neck, top of head, space between eyebrows, area between nose and upper lip and spot just below lower lip.
4 Stand up.

Points to remember
● *After squatting and sitting down peep around and scratch yourself like a monkey, then massage the specific points numerous times.*

CRANE PLAY

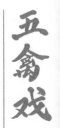

WING-FLAPPING TO THE LEFT

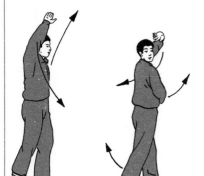

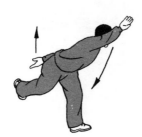

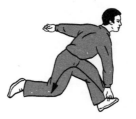

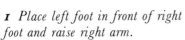

1 *Place left foot in front of right foot and raise right arm.*
2 *Drop right arm and hold it in front of abdomen, palm down; at same time raise left arm, palm up.*

3 *Lean forward and stretch right leg behind back, balancing body on left foot; at same time cross arms and stretch right arm forward and left arm back.*

4 *Touch left foot with right hand and stretch right hand toward back.*
5 *Touch left foot with right hand and stretch right hand toward back. Turn 45 degrees to the left, put right foot down and stand naturally.*

WING-FLAPPING TO THE RIGHT

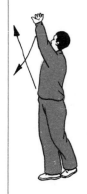

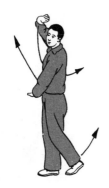

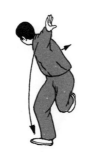

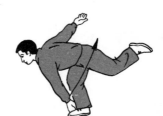

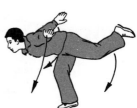

Repeat steps 1–5 of Wing-flapping to the left, but in opposite direction.

Points to remember
● *Stretch arms to full extent.*
● *When balancing body, keep steady, look straight ahead, relax shoulders and waist and breathe naturally.*

TURNING AND LOOKING BACK TO THE LEFT

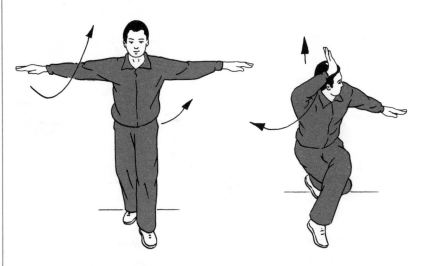

1 Step forward to right with left foot and stretch arms to side.

2 Lean forward and squat with right knee bent behind left knee; at same time bend right arm at level of head, palm up and stretch left arm toward back, eyes looking at left hand.

3 Return to position in Step *1*.
4 Step forward with right foot, drop arms and stand naturally.

TURNING AND LOOKING BACK TO THE RIGHT

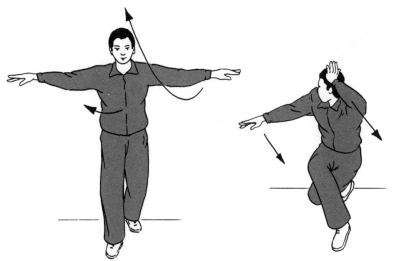

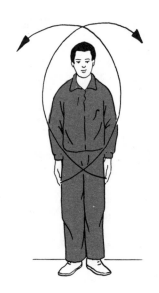

Repeat steps 1–4 of Turning and looking back to the left, but in opposite direction.

Points to remember
● *When squatting and turning to look back, keep one arm low and the other high; turn head back as far as possible and support bent knee with knee in front.*

SOARING

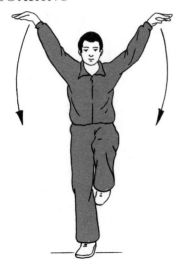

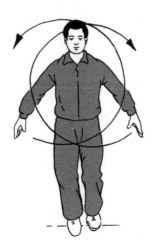

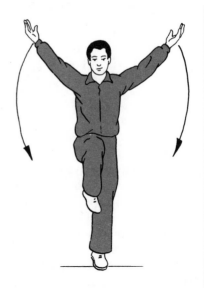

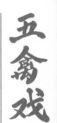

1 Following lines of step 4 of Turning and looking back to the right, cross arms in front of chest and raise them high like wings; at same time lift left knee.

2 Lower arms gradually and return left foot to ground.

3 Cross arms in front of chest and stretch them up like wings, palms up; at same time lift right knee.
4 Lower arms slowly and return right foot to ground.

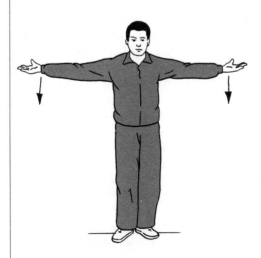

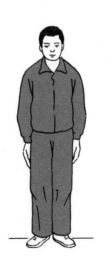

5 Raise arms to shoulder level, palms up and lower them; at same time stamp left or right foot once and return immediately to standing to attention position.

Points to remember
● *Move in coordinated fashion throughout exercise and imitate the graceful manner of a crane soaring high in the sky.*
● *Lift arms up when only one foot is on ground and lower them when both feet are on ground.*

INTERNAL
FORMS OF EXERCISE
PRINCIPLES

The internal forms of exercise, which emphasize slow movements and tranquillity of mind, have a completely different emphasis to the external forms of exercise. The most popular of all internal exercises is taiji shadow boxing, known in China as taijiquan. This is included here as well as taiji swordplay and the taiji duet.

The underlying principle of the internal exercises is the idea that action follows thought. An example of this is in the starting position, where the slow raising of arms occurs only after the thought of raising arms has occurred. All internal exercises are controlled by such consciousness and one must therefore be quiet and calm before beginning each exercise and then apply one's total concentration.

Relaxation is all-important. Muscles and joints should be relaxed to such a degree that all rigidity disappears. The torso should be kept upright with arms held in a rounded manner and legs bent or curved as required. Special attention must be paid to balance as one moves from one position to another and natural breathing is essential. The basic rule of 'up, inhale; down, exhale' naturally coordinates breathing with action. In the starting position, for example, the raising of the arms causes you to breathe in and the lowering of the arms to breathe out.

There are several distinguishing features of the internal forms of exercise. Lightness and suppleness characterize them all. Taijiquan should be done slowly and smoothly as the movements are in accord with the natural motions of the human body. After exercising one should feel relaxed and refreshed rather than exerted, and it is therefore especially suitable for the elderly, the infirm and sufferers of chronic diseases.

Continuity is important. Taijiquan from beginning to end should be a smooth, uninterrupted flow of movement. Movements of arms and hands in curves and arcs should follow the natural curves of your joints. This ensures an even exertion of each part of the body.

Finally, taijiquan requires a close coordination of the upper and lower parts of the body. Taijiquan also calls for harmony between inner and outer body movements and you must be aware of your breathing. Each movement involves the whole body, with the waist and back initiating the movement of your limbs. Such well-coordinated movements automatically eliminate any rigidity and disjointedness.

Pay special attention to certain parts of the body while doing these exercises. Move your head naturally with your torso, keep your chin in and mouth closed with your tongue resting gently behind your upper teeth, and breathe through your nose. Eyes should follow the hand that is in front and your neck should be neither too stiff nor too relaxed. Your chest should be pulled in and your shoulders should be kept low.

Gravity acts through your legs giving you firm contact with the ground, as can be seen by the constant shifting of weight from one leg to the other. Knee joints should be relaxed throughout, and even when told to keep legs straight the knee joints should never be locked. When advancing always touch the ground with your heel first and when retreating put your toe down first. The sinking of shoulders and lowering of elbows is especially important as, when these two joints are relaxed, arms and wrists become naturally curved and fingers naturally spread.

太极拳运动
TAIJI SHADOW BOXING

This simplified form of taiji shadow boxing, also known as taijiquan, was created by The Chinese National Sports Committee and has proved to be very popular with beginners and those who are pressed for time. Beginning with easy movements it gradually becomes more difficult and eliminates the repetitive movements of the conventional taijiquan (88 movements) while retaining its essence and distinctive techniques. It is composed of 24 movements, each with its own title, divided into eight groups and may be practiced as a whole or in sections. Make sure that you begin each movement in a north-facing position.

THE FIRST SECTION
Preparation
Parting of wild horse mane
White crane flaps its wings
THE SECOND SECTION
Brushing the knee
Strumming the lute
Curving back arms to left and right
THE THIRD SECTION
Grasping the bird's tail to the left
Grasping the bird's tail to the right
THE FOURTH SECTION
Single whip
Waving hands in the clouds
Single whip

THE FIFTH SECTION
Patting the horse
Kicking with the right heel
Striking ears with both fists
Kicking with the left heel
THE SIXTH SECTION
Sweeping down to left on one leg
Sweeping down to right on one leg
THE SEVENTH SECTION
Passing the shuttle to left and right
Needle at sea bottom
Dodge with the arm
THE EIGHTH SECTION
Turn to strike, parry and punch
Withdraw and push
Crossing arms
Conclusion

One must however always remember that taijiquan is essentially one continuous movement from beginning to end. The phrase 'at the same time' constantly appears and this is because in taijiquan all movements of the limbs and body are simultaneous and coordinated and cannot be separated and done individually. Each illustration is the continuation of the one before and is followed by the one after. The arrows must be studied carefully and the whole exercise will become easier if you can visualize a continuous flow of motion.

THE FIRST SECTION

PREPARATION

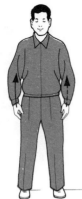 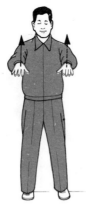 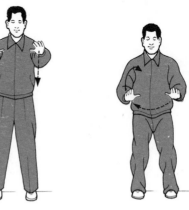

1 Stand to attention. Step to left so that feet are shoulder-width apart, relax arms and hold them by side. Keep head and neck up, pull abdomen in and look straight ahead.

2 Lower shoulders and slowly raise arms to shoulder level, palms down.
3 Lower elbows and wrists so that hands are upright.

4 Keep torso straight, bend knees and press hands down lightly; lower elbows toward knees.

PARTING OF WILD HORSE MANE

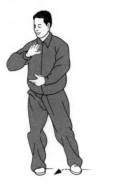 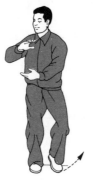 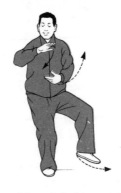 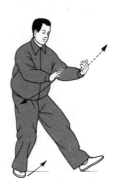 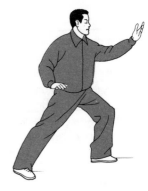

1 Turn torso slightly to right and put weight on right leg; at same time lift right hand, palm down, to chest level, and move left hand to right, palm up, and position hands as though holding a ball.

2 Move left foot, with heel raised, to right and keep eyes on right hand.
3 Turn torso slightly to left and step to left with left foot and with right leg straight, bend left knee.

4–5 At same time move left hand up to eye level, palm up, elbow slightly bent, and right hand down to waist level, palm down, elbow slightly bent; keep eyes on left hand.

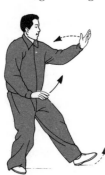 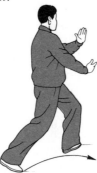 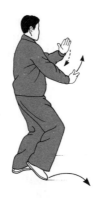 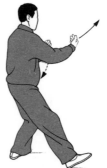 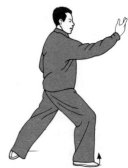

6 Slowly move torso back, shift weight to right leg and lift left toes off ground.
7 Move torso forward and to left, shifting weight to left leg; at same time draw left hand back toward

chest, palm down, move right palm up and position hands as though holding a ball.
8 Bring right foot next to left foot, lift right heel off ground and keep eyes on left hand.

9–10 Move right foot forward to right and keeping left leg straight, bend right knee and repeat steps 4–5, but in opposite direction.

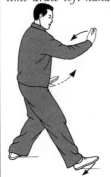 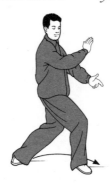 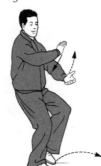 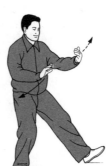 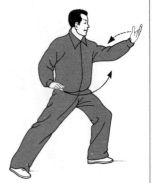

11–15 Repeat steps 1–5.

WHITE CRANE FLAPS ITS WINGS

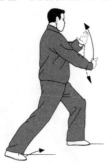
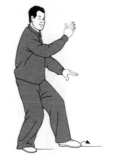
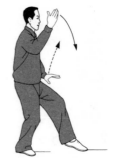

1 Turn torso slightly to left, lower left hand, palm down, and move right hand forward in a curve, palm up, and position hands as though holding a ball; keep eyes on left hand.

2 Move right foot half a step forward and shift weight back to right leg; at same time raise right hand to eye level, press down with left hand and turn torso to right.

3 Move left foot forward, lift heel off ground and turn torso slightly to left; raise right hand to level of forehead, drop left hand, palm down, by left hip and look ahead.

THE SECOND SECTION

BRUSHING THE KNEE

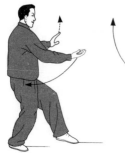
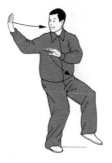
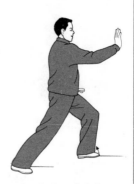

1–3 Turn torso slightly to left and then to right, lower right hand and pass it along right hip before raising it in a curve to eye level; at same time move left hand up, then down in a curve to front of chest; at same time point toes of left foot toward ground and keep eyes on right hand.

4–5 Turn torso to left, step to left with left foot and keeping right leg straight, bend left leg; at same time as turning torso push right hand forward at nose level, brush left hand across left knee and hold it by left hip, palm down; keep eyes on fingers of right hand.

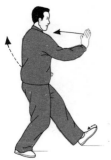
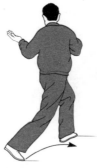
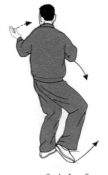
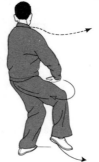
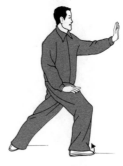

6–7 Bend right knee slowly, shift weight onto right leg and lift toes of left foot off ground. Turn torso to left and shift weight to left leg.
8 Bring right foot next to left foot and point toes of right foot toward ground; at same time turn left palm up and move it out to left. Follow turning of torso with right hand and bring it to right side of chest, palm down; keep eyes on left hand.

9–10 Repeat steps 4–5, but in opposite direction. ▶.

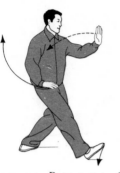
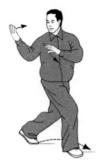
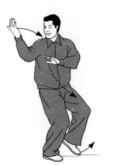
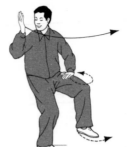
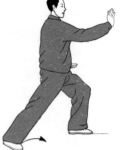

11–13 *Repeat steps 6–8, but in opposite direction.*

14–15 *Repeat steps 4–5.*

STRUMMING THE LUTE

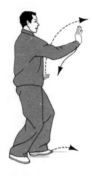
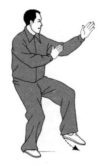
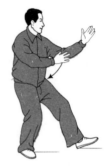

1–3 *Take half a step forward with right foot and lower torso, shifting weight onto right leg. Turn torso 90 degrees to right, lift left leg, move it forward and put it*

down with its toes off ground and knee slightly bent; at same time bring left hand up and forward to nose level, palm facing right, arm slightly bent, and draw right hand

back to face inside of left elbow, palm facing left and keep eyes on left thumb.

CURVING BACK ARMS TO LEFT AND RIGHT

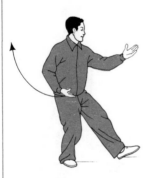
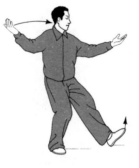
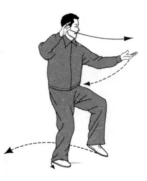
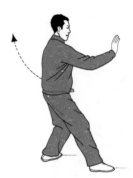

1–2 *Turn torso to right and draw right hand back and up in a curve with palm up and arm slightly bent. At same time turn left palm up, keep eyes to right as you turn torso*

and then turn to look at left hand. **3–4** *Bend right elbow, push right hand forward, palm facing front; bend left elbow and draw left hand back to waist, palm up. At same*

time lift left foot and take one step back, shift weight onto left leg, keeping eyes on right hand.

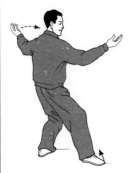
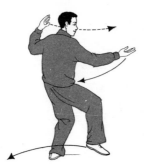
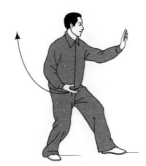
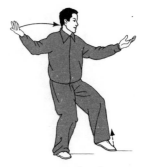

5 Turn torso slightly to left and raise left hand in a backward curve, palm up; at same time turn right

palm up, follow torso with eyes to left first and then turn to look at right hand.

6–8 Repeat steps 3–5, but in opposite direction.

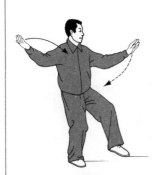
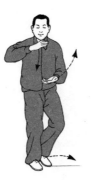
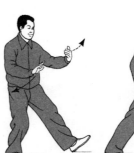
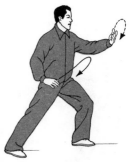

9–10 Repeat steps 3–4.
11 Repeat step 5.

12–13 Repeat steps 3–4, but in opposite direction.

THE THIRD SECTION

GRASPING THE BIRD'S TAIL TO THE LEFT

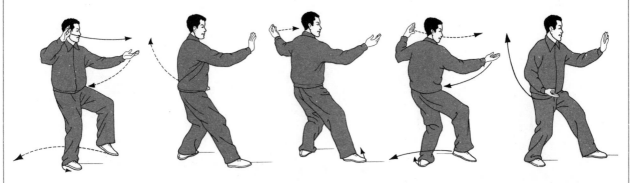

1 Turn torso slightly to right and draw right hand back and up in a curve. Relax left hand, palm down, and keep eyes on it.
2–3 Continue to turn torso to right, bring left hand down in a curve and hold it at rib cage, palm down,

bring right arm in front of chest, palm down and position hands as though holding a ball. At same time put weight on right leg, draw left foot in, toes pointing toward ground, and keep eyes on right hand.
4–5 Turn torso slightly to left,

step forward with left foot and keeping right leg straight, bend left knee; at same time move left forearm forward, palm facing body, and draw right hand back to hip, palm down. Keep eyes looking at left hand. ▶

太极拳运动

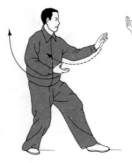
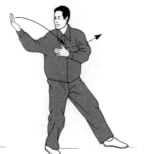
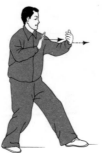

6–7 Turn left palm down and bring right palm up; turn torso to right and at same time move hands to right in a curve. Hold right hand at shoulder level, palm up, and bend

left arm in front of body, palm facing chest. Shift weight onto right leg and keep eyes on right hand.
8–9 Turn torso slightly to left, bend right elbow and bring right

hand toward left wrist, palms facing each other. Look at left wrist and keeping right leg straight, bend left leg and put weight on left leg.

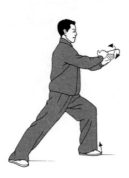
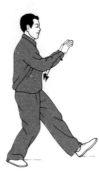
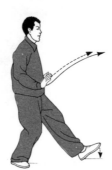
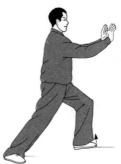

10–12 Turn left palm down and bring right hand over left wrist. Separate hands and hold them shoulder-width apart, palms down; at same time bend right knee, lower

torso and shift weight onto right leg with toes of left foot lifted off ground. Lower elbows, bring hands back to abdomen, and look ahead.

13 Shift weight forward slowly, keep right leg straight, bend left knee, push hands forward and look straight ahead.

GRASPING THE BIRD'S TAIL TO THE RIGHT

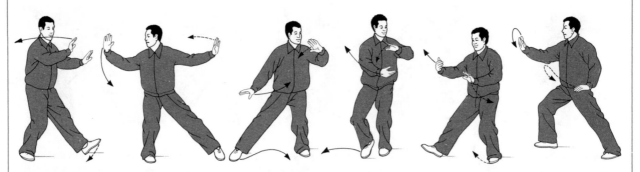

1 Lower torso, turn to right, bring right foot with you and shift weight to right leg; lift left toes off ground and turn them in.
2 Bring right hand behind back in a curve, follow movement with eyes.

3–4 Shift weight onto left leg, bring right hand down in a curve, hold it in front of left ribs, hold left hand in front of chest, palm down, and position hands as though holding a ball; at same time draw

right foot in with toes pointing to ground and keep eyes on left hand.
5–6 Repeat steps 4–5 of Grasping the bird's tail to the left, but in opposite direction.

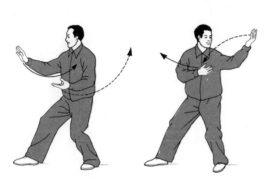

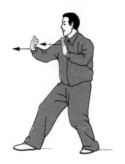

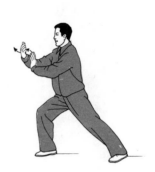

7–10 *Repeat steps 6–9 of Grasping the bird's tail to the left, but in opposite direction.*

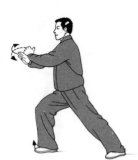

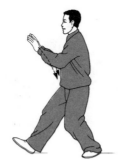

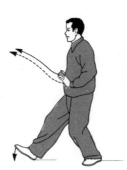

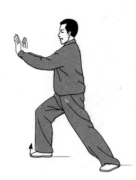

11–14 *Repeat steps 10–13 of Grasping the bird's tail to the left, but in opposite direction.*

THE FOURTH SECTION

SINGLE WHIP

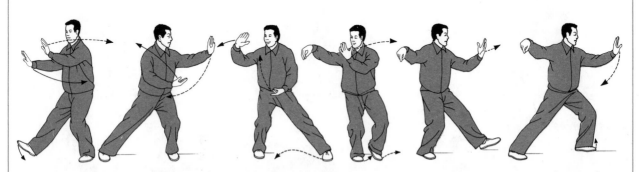

1 Lower torso, shift weight onto left leg and lift toes of right foot off ground and turn them in.

2 Turn torso to left, hold left hand at shoulder level, palm facing left, and right hand by left ribs, palm up; keep eyes on left hand.

3–4 Shift weight slowly to right leg while turning torso to right and drawing left foot in with only toes touching ground; at same time move right hand up in a curve to right at shoulder level, close fingers round thumb loosely and hang hand down from wrist joint. Pass left hand in front of abdomen to front of right shoulder. Keep eyes on left palm.

5–6 Turn torso to left, step forward with left foot and keeping left leg straight, bend right leg and shift weight onto left leg. At same time push left palm out, arm slightly bent, and keep eyes on left hand.

75

WAVING HANDS IN THE CLOUDS

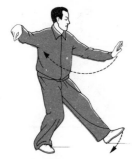 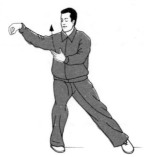 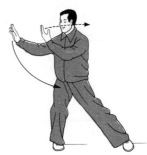

1 *Return weight to right leg and gradually turn torso to right with left toes raised and turning in.*

2-3 *Pass left hand in front of abdomen, move it up in a curve and hold it in front of right shoulder; at*

same time unhook right hand and turn palm up to face out, keeping eyes on left palm.

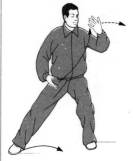 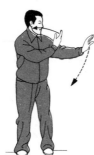 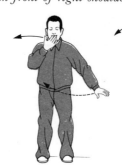 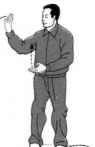 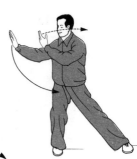

4-6 *Turn torso slowly to left, shift weight to left leg and draw right foot in so that it is parallel with the left foot; at same time move left hand in front of face to left, palm facing out, and bring right hand*

down in a curve and up to front of left shoulder, with eyes on right palm.
7-8 *Turn torso to right and keeping weight on right leg, stretch left leg over to left; at same time*

wave right hand to right, palm facing out, and move left hand down in a curve and up to front of right shoulder, keeping eyes on front of left shoulder.

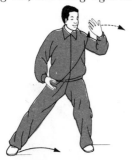 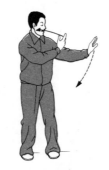 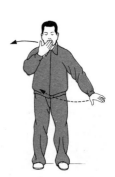

9-11 *Repeat steps 4-6.*

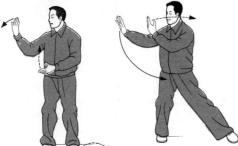 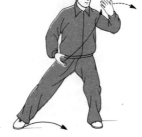 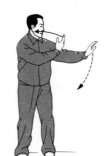 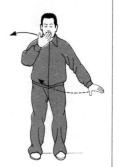

12-13 *Repeat steps 7-8.* **14-16** *Repeat steps 4-6.*

SINGLE WHIP

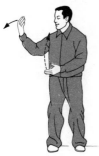 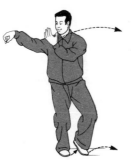 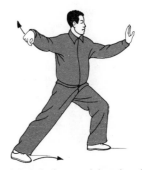

1–2 Turn torso to right and follow movement with right hand; at same time pass left hand in front of abdomen and move it up in a curve to front of right shoulder, keeping eyes on left palm. Close fingers of

right hand round thumb and hang hand from wrist joint. Shift weight to right leg and lift left heel so that toes remain touching ground.
3–4 Turn torso gradually to left, keep left hand at eye level, step to

left with left foot and keeping left leg straight, bend right knee. Shift weight onto left leg and while continuing to turn torso to left, turn left palm to push outward, forming a "single whip" position.

THE FIFTH SECTION

PATTING THE HORSE

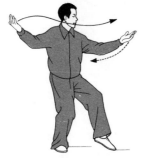 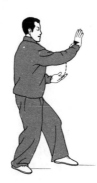

1 Take half a step forward with right foot and gradually shift weight back to right leg. Open right hand and turn both palms up, elbows slightly bent; at same time lift left

heel off ground and turn torso slightly to right.
2 Turn torso slightly to left, bring right hand past right ear and push forward, keeping fingers at eye level;

at same time draw left hand back to waist, palm up, and step forward with left foot, heel raised off ground, keeping eyes on right hand.

KICKING WITH THE RIGHT HEEL

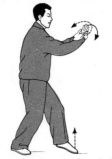 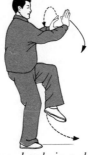 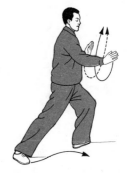

1 Cross wrists by passing left hand, palm up, over right hand.

2–3 Uncross hands in a downward motion, palms down, and at same time raise left leg and step out to

left. Keep right leg straight, bend left leg and shift weight forward. ▶

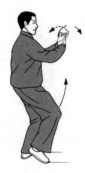 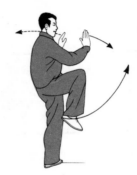 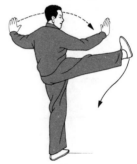

4 Move hands up in a curve, palms up, and cross wrists in front of chest with right hand on outside and palms facing in; at same time draw right

foot in and point toes to ground.
5–6 Spread arms out to sides, elbows slightly bent and palms facing out; at same time raise right

knee and slowly straighten leg; kick with right heel and keep eyes on right hand.

STRIKING EARS WITH BOTH FISTS

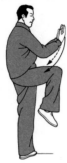 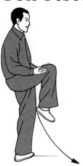 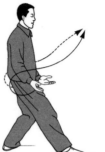 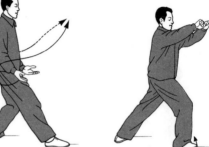

1–2 Draw right leg back with knee still raised; at same time bring left hand forward next to right hand, drop hands beside right knee, palms up, and look ahead.

3–4 Put right foot forward and step forward. Shift weight gradually to right leg, which should be bent, and keep left leg straight; at same time clench fists slowly and lower

them first to sides and then up and forward at eye level. Keep fists facing each other at a distance of 10–20 cm (4–8 in) and keep eyes on right fist.

KICKING WITH THE LEFT HEEL

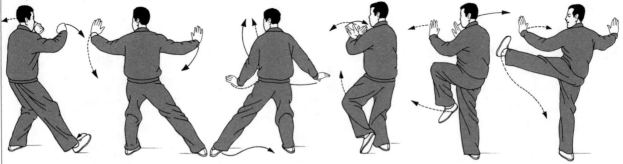

1 Bend left knee, shift weight to left leg and turn torso to left, toes of right foot raised and turned in.
2 At same time unclench fists and spread arms to sides, palms facing forward, eyes looking at left hand.

3–4 Shift weight onto right leg and draw left foot in, toes pointing to ground; at same time move hands down and up in a curve and cross wrists in front of chest with left hand on outside, palms facing in.

5–6 Spread arms out to sides, elbows slightly bent and palms facing out; at same time raise left knee and straighten leg slowly, kicking with left heel, eyes looking at left hand.

THE SIXTH SECTION

SWEEPING DOWN TO LEFT ON ONE LEG

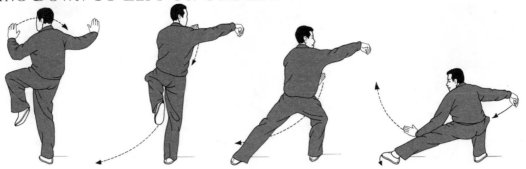

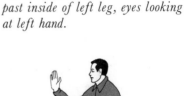

1–2 Draw left leg back with knee still raised and turn torso to right; at same time hook right hand by bending wrist and move left hand up in a curve and down to front of

right shoulder, palm facing in and eyes looking at right hand.
3 Bend right knee slowly, lower left leg and stretch it out to left.
4 While squatting down on right

leg move left hand down in a curve, past inside of left leg, eyes looking at left hand.

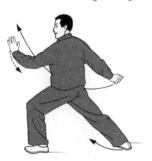

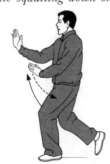

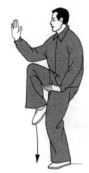

5 Shift weight forward to left leg, which should be bent, and keep right leg straight; turn left toes out and right toes in as much as possible. At same time continue to stretch left

hand forward, palm upright, and lower right hand, which should be hooked, and keep eyes on left hand.
6–7 Raise right knee slowly and stand on left leg; at same time raise

right hand to eye level with elbow bent just above right knee and palm facing left. Lower left hand to hip, palm down, and look at right hand.

SWEEPING DOWN TO RIGHT ON ONE LEG

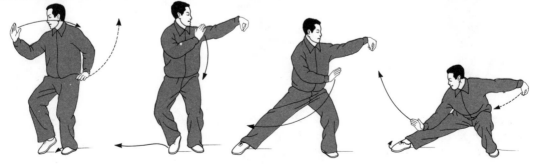

1–2 Place right foot in front of left foot, keeping right heel off ground, and pivoting on ball of left foot turn body to left. At same time raise left

arm, hook left hand and move right hand to front of left shoulder, palm facing in and eyes on left hand.

3–4 Repeat steps 3–4 of Sweeping down to left on one leg, but in opposite direction. ▶

太极拳运动

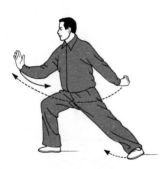

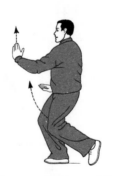

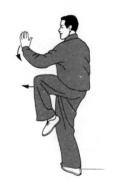

5 Repeat step 5 of Sweeping down to left on one leg, but in opposite direction.

6–7 Repeat steps 6–7 of Sweeping down to left on one leg, but in opposite direction.

THE SEVENTH SECTION

PASSING THE SHUTTLE TO LEFT AND RIGHT

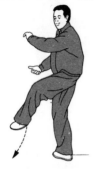

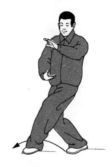

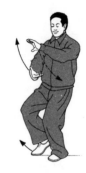

1–2 Turn body slightly to left and place left foot in front of right foot. Squat and lift right heel; at same

time position hands in front of chest as though holding a ball, left hand above right hand.

3 Draw right foot next to left foot with only toes touching ground and keep eyes on left arm.

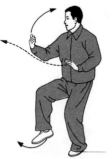

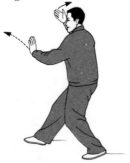

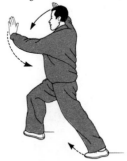

4–6 Turn body to right, step forward with right foot and keeping left leg straight, bend right knee; at

same time lift right hand and hold it to right side of forehead, palm up. Lower left hand and push it

forward until it reaches eye level, palm facing forward; keep eyes on left hand.

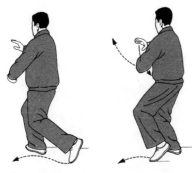 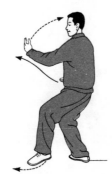 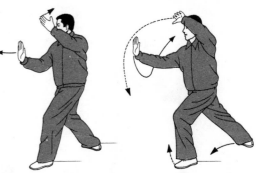

7–8 *Shift weight slightly back so that toes of right foot turn out. Put weight on right leg and draw left foot beside right foot, left heel*

raised; at same time position hands in front of chest as though holding a ball, right hand above left hand, and keep eyes on right arm.

9–11 *Repeat steps 4–6, but in opposite direction.*

NEEDLE AT SEA BOTTOM

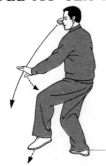 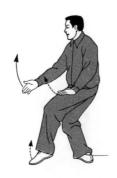

1–2 *Take half a step forward with right foot, shift weight to right leg, lift left foot and point toes to ground; at same time turn body*

slightly to right and move right hand down in a curve and up to side of right ear. Turn body to left, drop right hand forward, palm facing

left; at same time lower left hand forward, then down in a curve and rest it at side of left hip, palm down; keep eyes on right hand.

DODGE WITH THE ARM

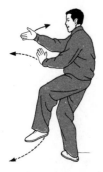 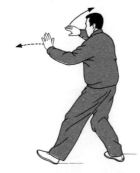 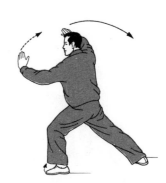

1 *Turn torso slightly to right and step forward with left foot, keep right leg straight and bend left knee.*
2 *At same time raise right hand,*

bend elbow and hold hand at right side of forehead, palm up.
3 *At same time lift left hand and push it forward at chest level with*

palm facing front; keep eyes on left hand.

THE EIGHTH SECTION

TURN TO STRIKE, PARRY AND PUNCH

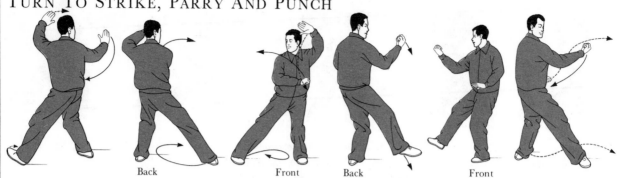

Back   Front   Back   Front

1 Lower torso, shift weight onto right leg and turn body to right with toes of left foot lifted off ground; at same time lift left hand and hold it in front of forehead with palm facing out.

2 Shift weight back to left leg, turn

body slightly to right and move right hand down in a curve and hold it in front of left rib cage, palm down; keep eyes looking to right.

3–4 Turn body to right, draw right leg back and step forward again; at same time flick right fist

over to right, crossing chest, palm up, and drop left hand beside hip, palm down. Drop right foot firmly on ground, its toes turned out, and keep eyes on right fist.

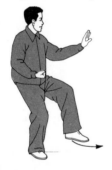

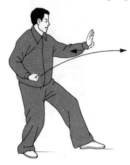

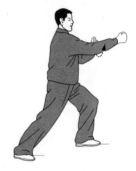

5–6 Shift weight onto right leg and step forward with left foot; at same time push forward with left hand and draw right fist back to waist,

palm up, eyes looking at left hand.
7 Keep right leg straight, bend left knee and punch forward with right fist, thumb facing up; hold inside of

right elbow with left hand, keeping eyes on right fist.

WITHDRAW AND PUSH

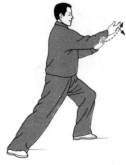

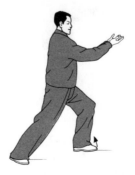

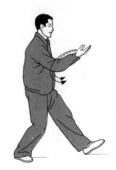

1–2 Stretch left hand out, passing it under right wrist, and unclench right fist so that palms face up.

3 Lower elbows slowly and draw hands back; at same time lower

torso, shift weight to right leg and lift toes of left foot off ground.

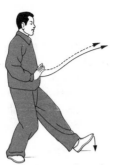

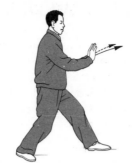

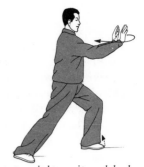

4–6 *Turn palms over and push forward with hands from abdomen*

up to shoulder level. At same time keeping right leg straight, bend left

leg, put weight on it and look straight ahead.

CROSSING ARMS

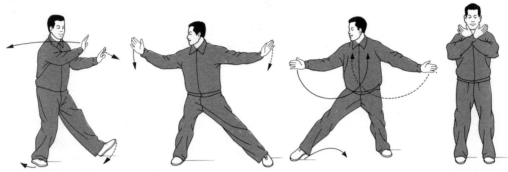

1–2 *Bend right knee, shift weight to right leg, lift left foot and turn toes in; at same time turn body to right and stretch right arm up so that palms are facing out. Bend*

elbows slightly and keep eyes on right hand.
3–4 *Shift weight slowly to left leg and draw right foot back so that it is parallel with left foot, but*

shoulder-width apart. At same time bring hands down and up to shoulder level and cross arms, right hand on outside, palms facing in, and look straight ahead.

CONCLUSION

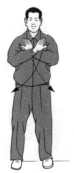

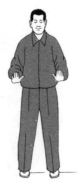

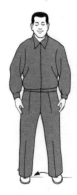

1–3 *Turn palms over to face out, slowly drop arms to side, palms facing down, and look straight*

ahead. When lowering arms relax whole body, breathe out slowly,

bring left foot next to right foot and stand straight.

太极劍

TAIJI SWORDPLAY

Taiji swordplay differs from other kinds of swordplay in that it is based on the principles of taijiquan and is therefore not a vigorous exercise and is suitable for the elderly. With the exception of the preparation position and conclusion, taiji swordplay contains 32 movements divided into four sections. The complete exercise when learnt lasts for about two to three minutes and can be practiced alone or in a group.

The Chinese terms for sword movements are used since no precise equivalents can be found in English.

THE BASICS

HOLDING SWORD IN LEFT HAND

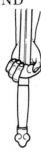

Hold guard with thumb pointing down, index finger stretched, and other fingers pointing up. Make sure that sword is close to body and parallel to left forearm with blade facing away from body.

HOLDING SWORD IN RIGHT HAND

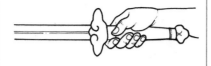

Hold handle with thumb and index finger, keep other three fingers in a more relaxed and flexible position and control movement of sword with base of palm. An alternative way to hold sword in right hand is to tighten middle finger, ring finger and thumb around handle and to relax index finger and little finger.

SWORD FINGERS

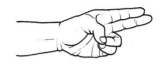

Whether holding sword in right or left hand, form sword fingers with hand that is not holding sword: stretch index and middle finger and bend little finger, thumb and ring finger into palm of hand.

PREPARATION

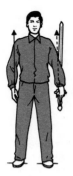 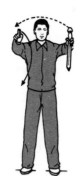 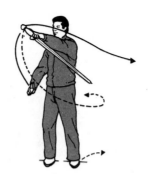 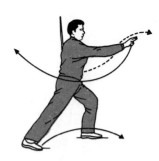

1 *Stand at ease, keep body straight with feet shoulder-width apart, toes pointing forward and arms hanging naturally. Hold sword, pointing straight up, in left hand, look straight ahead and relax shoulders.*
2 *Raise arms slowly to shoulder level, form right hand into sword fingers, palms of both hands facing down, and hold sword parallel to ground.*
3–4 *Turn torso slightly to right, shift weight to right leg; lower body, turn torso to left, lift leg, step to left and, keeping right leg straight, bend left knee. At same time move left hand to right and follow turning of torso downward in a curve to left; hold hand at left hip with sword pointing straight up. Simultaneously drop sword fingers, then bring them up and forward and point them straight ahead at eye level. Keep eyes on sword fingers.*

太
极
劍

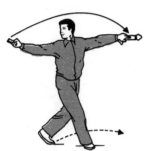

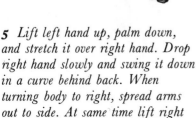

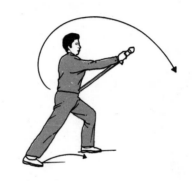

5 Lift left hand up, palm down, and stretch it over right hand. Drop right hand slowly and swing it down in a curve behind back. When turning body to right, spread arms out to side. At same time lift right

leg and cross it over left leg. Keep knees bent with left heel off ground and keep eyes on sword fingers.
6 With right foot and left hand in position, step forward with left foot and, keeping right leg straight, bend

left knee; at same time turn torso to left and raise right hand formed into sword fingers over head to reach sword handle. Keep eyes on sword fingers.

THE FIRST SECTION

DIAN (TO POINT) WITH FEET TOGETHER

CI (TO THRUST) STANDING ON ONE FOOT

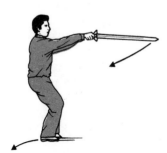

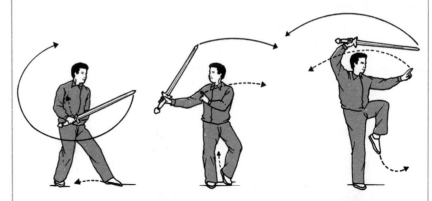

Hold sword in right hand and move it up and down in a curve. Point sword forward and take hold of right wrist with left hand formed into sword fingers; at same time bring right foot forward so that feet are together and bend knees; keep eyes on tip of sword.

Points to remember
● When moving sword up and down in a curve use only wrists and do not raise arms.
● When pointing sword concentrate on tip, keep shoulders relaxed and torso straight.

1–2 Step back with right foot and turn torso to right, then draw left foot back with heel off ground; at same time turn right wrist over and bring right hand over behind you, drawing a circle with tip of sword. Follow sword with left hand formed into sword fingers and rest them on right shoulder; keep eyes resting on tip of sword.

3 Turn torso to left, lift left knee and stand firmly on right foot. At same time raise right hand and pass sword over head with a thrusting movement. Stretch left hand, formed into sword fingers, forward and keep eyes on fingers.

Points to remember
● Do not pause in middle of movement.

SAO (TO SWEEP) FROM RIGHT TO LEFT

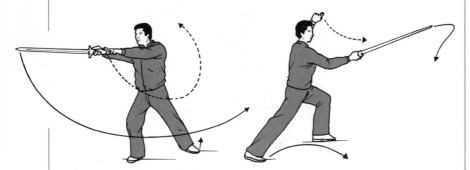

1 Turn torso to right and make a pi (chopping) movement, bringing sword back and behind to right and keep arm straight. Hold right wrist with left hand formed into sword fingers. At same time keeping left leg straight, bend right knee, lower left leg and stretch it backward; keep eyes on tip of sword.
2 Turn torso to left and swing left hand formed into sword fingers over and down and up in a curve and hold above head, palm facing up.

At same time sweep sword in same direction. While making sweeping movement and following turning of body, shift weight onto left foot and, keeping right leg straight, bend left knee; keep eyes on tip of sword.

Points to remember
● These two movements are continuous.
● When bending right or left knee keep torso upright.

DAI (TO TAKE THE LEAD) TO THE RIGHT

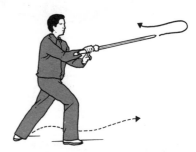

Lift right leg, step forward and, keeping left leg straight, bend right knee; at same time stretch right hand, turn sword-holding palm downward and slowly withdraw sword with elbow slightly bent in front of right ribs. Drop left hand formed into sword fingers to right wrist and keep eyes on tip of sword.

Points to remember
● Withdraw sword and bend right knee simultaneously.

DAI (TO TAKE THE LEAD) TO THE LEFT

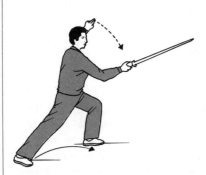

Stretch right hand forward, turn sword-holding palm upward and slowly withdraw sword with elbow slightly bent in front of left ribs; at same time bring left hand formed into sword fingers down past left ribs and up in a curve to left of forehead, palm up. At same time step forward with left foot and, keeping right leg straight, bend left knee; keep eyes on tip of sword.

PI (TO CHOP) STANDING ON ONE FOOT

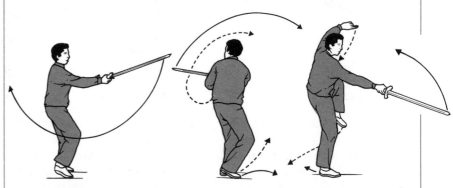

1 Bring right foot beside left foot, heel off ground, and drop left hand formed into sword fingers onto right wrist.
2 Turn body to left and bring sword back and behind in a curve to left, turning wrist up.
3 Swing left hand formed into sword fingers over head, palm up; at same time make a chopping movement with sword to right, step

forward with right foot and lift left knee-high, keep eyes on tip of sword.

Points to remember
● All movements are continuous.
● Eyes should follow tip of sword.
● Lift knee and make chopping movement simultaneously.

RETREAT AND CHOU (TO WHIP)

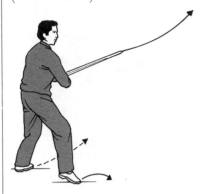

Drop left foot behind back, knee bent, and draw right foot back half a step, heel off ground; at same time make a whipping movement, bring your sword handle close to left ribs, tip of sword pointing outward. Drop left hand formed into sword fingers onto sword handle.

Points to remember
● *Draw right foot back and make whipping movement simultaneously.*
● *Keep torso upright.*

UPWARD CI (TO THRUST) ON ONE FOOT

Step forward with right foot and lift left knee high; at same time thrust sword up, palm up. Keep left hand formed into sword fingers on handle of sword and keep eyes on tip.

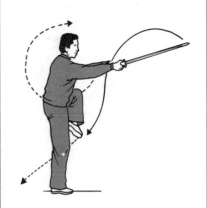

Points to remember
● *Stand firmly on one foot.*
● *Do not push chest forward.*

THE SECOND SECTION

DOWNWARD JIE (TO CUT)

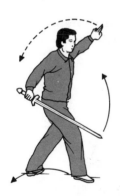

Drop left foot behind back and draw right foot slightly back, heel off ground; at same time following turning of body, first to left and then to right, make a downward cutting movement with sword, its tip at knee level. Bring left hand formed into sword fingers down and up in a curve to top left corner of forehead, palm up, and look straight ahead.

Points to remember
● *Move right foot and make cutting movement simultaneously.*
● *Turn body to right.*

CI (TO THRUST) TO THE LEFT

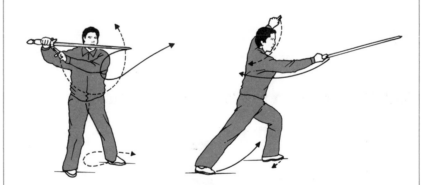

1–2 Step back with right foot, draw left foot back then step forward to left and, keeping right leg straight, bend left knee. At same time following movement of body bring sword to shoulder level, draw it back, lower it and make a forward thrusting movement to left, palm up; at same time drop left hand formed into sword fingers down in a curve to right, raise them in a curve to top left corner of forehead, palm up, and keep eyes on tip of sword.

Points to remember
● *When drawing sword back turn forearm out, when lowering sword turn forearm in, when thrusting sword from level of right hip turn forearm out.*

太极剑

TURN AROUND AND DAI
(TO TAKE THE LEAD)

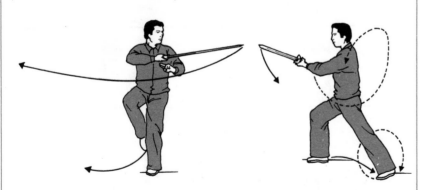

SHRINK BACK AND DAI
(TO TAKE THE LEAD)

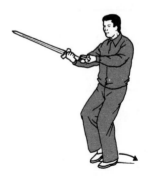

1 Pivoting on left heel, turn body to right and lift right foot to touch left leg; at same time draw right hand back to chest, palm up. Keep blade of sword parallel to ground, drop left hand formed into sword fingers to rest on right wrist and keep eyes on tip of sword.

2 Turn body to right, drop right foot to ground and, keeping left leg straight, bend right knee; at same time following turning of body, make a dai movement toward right with sword – exert force on outside of blade and turn tip of sword up and keep palm down. Rest left hand formed into sword fingers on right wrist and keep eyes on tip of sword.

Points to remember
● All movements must be smooth and coordinated.

Lift and lower left leg, draw right foot back next to left foot, heel off ground, while shifting weight onto left foot; at same time make a dai movement toward left with sword, palm up – exert force on outside of blade and turn tip of sword up. Move left hand formed into sword fingers down and back in a curve and then return them to rest on right wrist keeping eyes on tip of sword.

Points to remember
● Follow dai movement with body to left.

LIFTING KNEE AND HOLDING SWORD

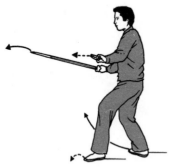

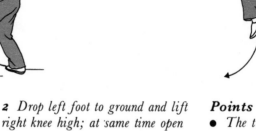

1 Step back with right foot and follow with left foot, heel off ground; at same time separate hands moving hand with sword to right and right hand formed into sword fingers to left, both palms down.

2 Drop left foot to ground and lift right knee high; at same time open left hand to hold right hand and bring sword handle toward chest, arms slightly bent, sword pointing forward and eyes looking ahead.

Points to remember
● The two movements are continuous.
● When standing on one leg, keep body upright.

HOP AND CI (TO THRUST)

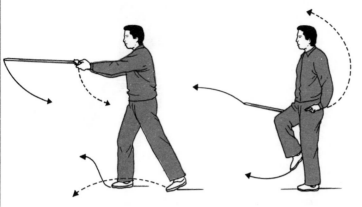

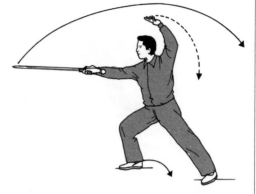

1 Lower right foot, shift weight forward; at same time thrust sword forward with force.
2 Stamp toes of right foot hard, step forward with left foot and quickly raise right heel to side of left leg; at same time separate and lower hands to sides, palms down,

left hand formed into sword fingers, eyes looking straight ahead.
3 Step forward with right foot and, keeping left leg straight, bend right knee; at same time thrust sword forward, palm up, eyes looking at tip of sword. Bring left hand formed into sword fingers over head

in a backward and upward curve, palm up.

Points to remember
● *Draw hands back a little before thrusting sword forward.*
● *Move feet quickly as though hopping.*

LIAO (TO PROVOKE) TO THE LEFT

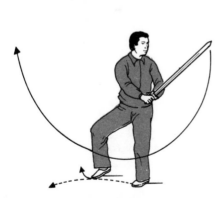

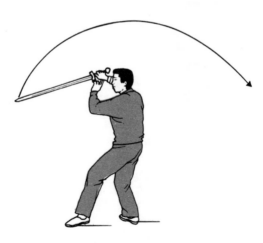

1–2 Turn torso to left and shift weight onto left leg. Draw right foot back half a step and, with weight shifted onto right leg, turn body to right and step forward with left foot, its heel off ground. At same time, following turning of

body, make a provocative movement – right forearm turned inward and palm facing outward – with sword in a curve down to left and then up in a curve to right. Stop sword handle at eye level and follow movement of right wrist with left

hand formed into sword fingers and keep eyes on tip of sword.

Points to remember
● *The whole movement is continuous and the liao movement should turn a full circle.*

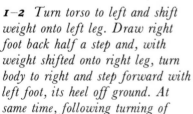

太极剑

LIAO (TO PROVOKE) TO THE RIGHT

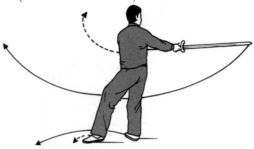

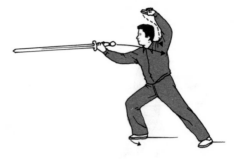

1 Turn torso to right and draw sword up and down to right in a curve, both palms facing out.
2 Put left foot down, step to left with right foot and, keeping left leg straight, bend right knee. At same time continue the provocative movement of sword down and up in a curve to left – turn right forearm out with palm facing out. Keep sword at shoulder level, raise left hand formed into sword fingers above head and keep eyes on tip of sword.

Points to remember
● Whole movement is continuous.
● Provocative movement should complete a whole circle.

THE THIRD SECTION

TURN LEFT AND CHOU (TO LASH)

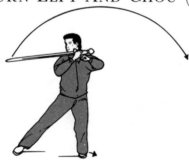

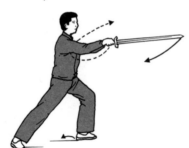

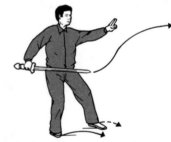

1 Turn body to left, shifting weight backward, straighten right leg and bend left knee slightly; at same time draw sword back to front of chest, with left hand formed into sword fingers touching right wrist.
2 Continue to turn to left with left knee bent and make a chopping movement to left with sword, keeping eyes on tip of sword.
3 Bend right knee slightly, shifting weight back to right leg and draw left foot back, heel off ground; at same time make a lashing movement, pulling sword back to right hip; draw left hand formed into sword fingers back to chest, stretch them forward again, keep eyes on fingers.

Points to remember
● Turn toes of right foot in before turning body.
● Bend right elbow toward chest before making chopping movement.

CI (TO THRUST) WITH FEET TOGETHER

Put left foot down, move right foot forward and stand straight with feet together; at same time open left hand to hold right hand and thrust sword forward, palms up, eyes looking at tip of sword.

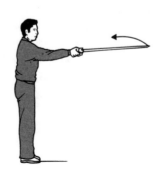

Points to remember
● Move feet and thrust sword simultaneously and keep arms slightly bent.

LAN (TO PARRY) TO THE LEFT

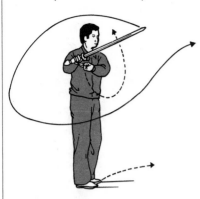 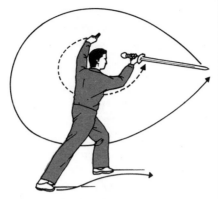

1 Pull sword back, keep left hand formed into sword fingers at right wrist and turn torso to right.
2 Follow turning of body to left and make a parrying movement with sword, drawing a backward, downward and forward curve to left – right forearm turned outward. Raise left hand formed into sword fingers above head; at same time step forward to left with left foot and, keeping right leg straight, bend left knee and keep eyes on movement of sword.

Points to remember
● Turn body first to right then to left following movement of sword.

LAN (TO PARRY) TO THE RIGHT

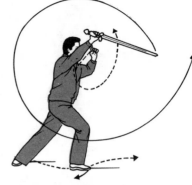

Shift weight slightly backward while turning torso to left with toes of left foot slanting out, then turn torso to right, step forward with right foot and, keeping left leg straight, bend right knee; at same time parry with sword to left in a downward and forward curve – turn right forearm in, palm facing out; at same time return left hand formed into sword fingers to right wrist and keep eyes on movement of sword.

太极剑

LAN (TO PARRY) TO THE LEFT

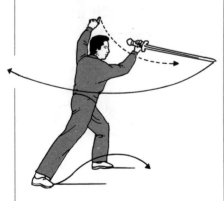

Shift weight slightly backward while turning toes of right foot out, step forward with left foot and, keeping right leg straight, bend left knee and turn torso to left; at same time parry with sword in a backward, downward and forward curve – turn right forearm out and raise left hand formed into sword fingers above head.

STEP UP AND CI (TO STAB)

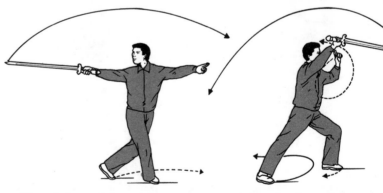

1 Turn body to right and cross right leg over to left, lifting heel off ground; at same time lower tip of sword, drop left hand formed into sword fingers to right wrist, spread arms out and make a stabbing movement with sword to right, palm facing forward, eyes following tip of sword.
2 Turn body to left, step forward with left foot and, keeping right leg straight, bend left knee; at same time bring tip of sword down in a curve to left with right forearm turned in and palm facing out; rest left hand formed into sword fingers on right wrist and keep eyes on tip of sword.

Points to remember
● Two movements are continuous..
● When bending left knee do not lean forward too much.

TURN BACK AND PI (TO CHOP)

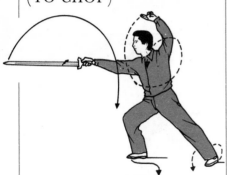

Shift weight onto right foot while turning toes of left foot in, lift right leg and shift weight onto left leg. Turn body to right, step forward with right foot and, keeping left leg straight, bend right knee; at same time make a chopping movement

with sword in same direction as body is turning; lift left hand formed into sword fingers above head in an upward and downward curve. Keep eyes on tip of sword.

DIAN (TO POINT) WITH RIGHT TOES POINTING FORWARD

Lift left foot while turning torso to left, put left foot down and lift right foot up and put it down in front of left foot with heel off ground; at same time draw sword up in a curve and point it forward and down. Form left hand into sword fingers and bring them round in a circle to rest on right wrist; keep eyes on tip of sword.

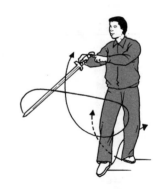

Points to remember
● When pointing forward exert force on wrist and tip of sword and the movement should be simultaneous with landing of right foot on ground.

THE FOURTH SECTION

TUO (TO HOLD) STANDING ON ONE FOOT

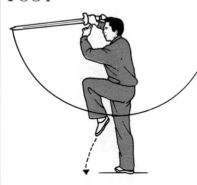

Bring right foot behind left foot and, pivoting on balls of both feet, turn body to right and raise left knee; at same time draw circle with sword (left, down and up) and hold sword up to right slightly above level of head. Form left hand into sword fingers, hold it at right wrist and look straight ahead.

Points to remember
● Lift left knee and hold sword up at same time.
● Stand firmly on right leg.

GUA (TO HANG) AND PI (TO CHOP)

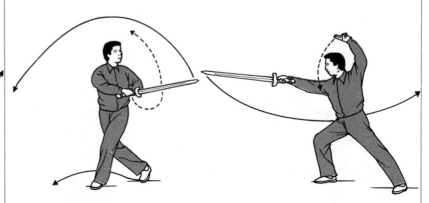

1 Drop left foot to side and turn body to left, knees crossed and bent, right heel off ground; at same time make a hanging movement with sword to rear, keep left hand formed into sword fingers at right wrist and follow tip of sword with eyes.
2 Make a chopping movement with sword toward right; lift left hand formed into sword fingers above head

and at same time step forward with right foot and, keeping left leg straight, bend right knee, keeping eyes on tip of sword.

Points to remember
● The two movements are continuous; turn body first to left and then to right.

LIAO (TO PROVOKE) AND PI (TO CHOP)

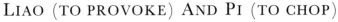

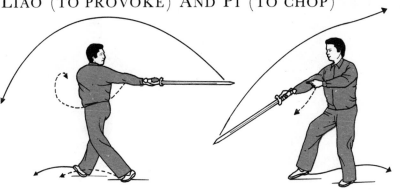

1 Shift weight slightly backward and turn body to left, knees crossed, and lift left heel off ground; at same time make a provocative movement with sword in a downward curve and up to the right; drop left hand formed into sword fingers to right shoulder and keep eyes on tip of sword.

2 Step forward with left foot, turn body to left then step forward with right foot, its heel off ground; at

same time make a forward chopping movement with sword first backward then forward, keeping tip of sword level with knee. Move left hand formed into sword fingers down in a curve and up to rest on right forearm; keep eyes on tip of sword.

Points to remember
● *The two movements are continuous and do not pause in the middle.*

STEP BACK AND JI (TO STRIKE)

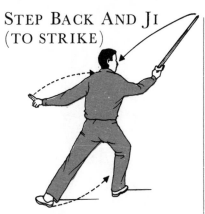

太极劍

Turn body to right and take a large step back with right foot and, keeping left leg straight, bend right knee; at same time make a striking movement with sword back and upward following turning of body and hold tip of sword above eye level. Point left hand formed into sword fingers toward left, keep eyes on tip of sword.

Points to remember
● *Step back with right foot then straighten left leg.*

STEP FORWARD AND CI (TO THRUST)

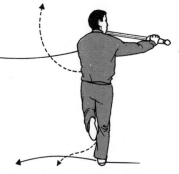

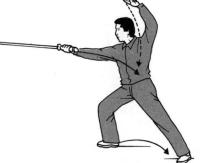

1 Lift left leg and bring it down close to right leg; at same time turn right palm over and bring sword to front of right shoulder, pointing to left; bring left hand formed into sword fingers to right shoulder and look straight ahead.

2 Turn round and toward left, place left foot on ground, step forward with right foot and, keeping left leg straight, bend right knee; at same time as turning body thrust sword forward with force, palm up. Raise left hand formed into sword fingers above head.

RETREAT AND CHOU (TO WHIP)

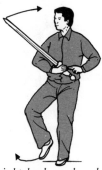

Shift weight backward and draw right foot back beside left foot, its heel off ground; at same time bend right elbow and draw back sword, palm facing in and sword handle at left ribs. Drop left hand formed into sword fingers onto handle and keep eyes on tip of sword.

Points to remember
● *Draw back right foot and sword at the same time.*

太
极
剑

Ma (to swipe) With Body Revolving

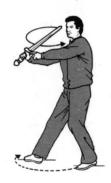
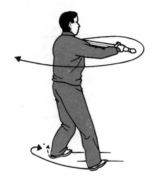
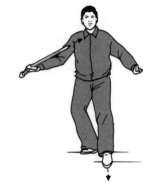

1 Lift right foot and step forward with toes turned out; at same time turn torso slightly to right and stretch arms out so that sword is positioned in front of chest.
2–3 Shift weight onto right leg and keep turning to right; move left foot in front of right foot, toes pointing toward each other; pivoting on ball

of left foot, continue to turn body to right until right foot is a step behind left foot; draw left foot back half a step, toes pointing toward ground. At same time following revolving of body, make a sweeping movement with sword parallel to ground and separate hands with palms facing down.

Points to remember
● All movements should be done in a continuous flow.
● Keep torso straight throughout.

Ci (to stab) Straight Forward

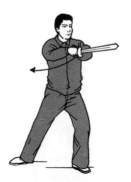

Take half a step forward with left foot and, keeping right leg straight, bend left knee; at same time make a stabbing movement with sword, thrusting it straight forward. Keep left hand formed into sword fingers resting on right wrist and look straight ahead.

Points to remember
● Bend left leg and make stabbing movement at same time.

Conclusion

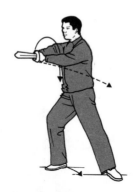
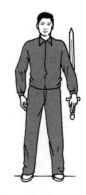

1 Shift weight backward and turn body to right; at same time draw back sword, palm facing in, and put left hand on hand guard, palm facing right palm. Keep eyes on sword.
2 Turn body to left, shifting weight onto left leg, and bring right foot parallel with left foot, but

shoulder-width apart; at same time take hold of sword with left hand and drop it naturally to side, keeping blade of sword parallel with forearm. Draw right hand back and up in a curve and hang it by side. Relax whole body and look ahead.

太极推手
THE TAIJI DUET

The taiji duet, also known as taiji tuishou, is a highly developed form of taiji shadow boxing and it requires two people to exercise together, thereby creating an element of confrontation. While practicing, the two may learn from each other and improve their own basic techniques of taiji shadow boxing. Beginners may take up taiji shadow boxing and the taiji duet at the same time.

Start with the basic single-hand techniques, go on to the two-hand techniques and tuishou on fixed feet and finish with tuishou on movable feet. Beginners must be very patient and move from the easy exercises to the more difficult gradually.

As in all forms of taiji the movements are fluid and continuous and body, arms and legs must be relaxed. Partners should not come into direct conflict with each other, nor should they avoid each other. The basic principle of the taiji duet is to take advantage of an onward force and to neutralize it: when **A** advances, **B** retreats; when **A** retreats, **B** advances, and so on.

Study the illustrations carefully and follow the arrows for movements of hands and feet. The figure on the left is **A** and the figure on the right is **B**.

BASIC MOVEMENTS

PREPARATION
Stand facing each other with bodies completely relaxed. Measure distance between each other by raising arms and touching each other's fists.

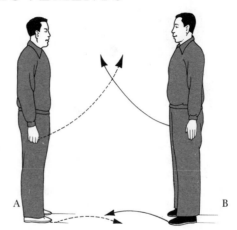

BASIC SINGLE-HAND TECHNIQUES

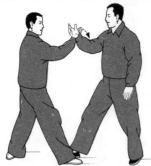
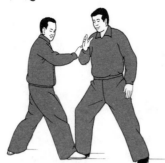
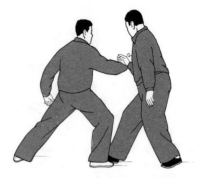

Starting position *Both half turn to left and step forward with right foot so that insides of feet face each other at a distance of 4–8 in (10–20 cm). Both raise right hand with elbow bent and backs of hands lightly touching each other and make sure that the counter-force is neither* too strong nor too weak. Let left hand hang naturally.
*1 **A** turn over right hand, using palm to push **B**'s wrist; at same time **A** bend right knee, shift weight forward a little and try to reach right-hand side of **B**'s chest with right hand.*

*2 **B** do not resist **A**'s pressure and fold arm toward chest; at same time bend left knee and shift weight back a little, turn torso to right and divert **A**'s hand away from chest with right palm.* ▶

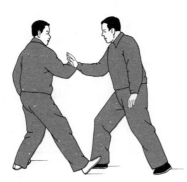

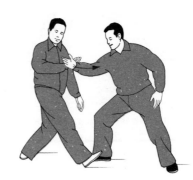

3 *B turn over right hand, use palm to push A's wrist and try to reach right side of A's chest.*

4 *A do not resist B's pressure and bend left knee, shift weight backward and turn torso to right,*

using right palm to ward off B's right hand.

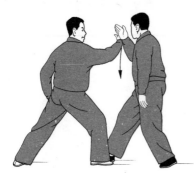

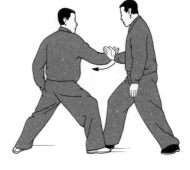

5 *Return to starting position. A turn right hand over, using palm to push B's wrist forward and up and try to reach for B's face; at same time bend right knee and shift*

weight forward a little. B do not resist A's force and take advantage of situation by lifting arm. Bend left knee slightly, shift weight back a little, turn torso to right and

divert A's hand away to right of his head.

6 *B slowly press right hand down and forward and try to reach for A's right ribs.*

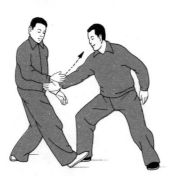

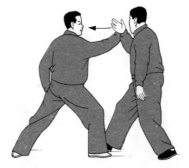

7 *A do not resist B's force and withdraw right arm; at same time bend left knee, shift weight back a*

little, turn torso to right and divert B's hand away to right of his body.

8 *A reach for B's face with right*

hand and B turn right to divert A's hand away to right of his head.

太極推手

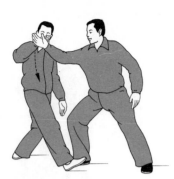
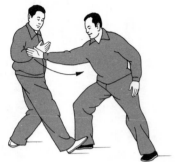

9–10 B take advantage of the situation by reaching for **A**'s face. **A** bend left leg a little, turn right to neutralize **B**'s force, continue to push down and forward with palm and reach for **B**'s right ribs. Repeat exercise many times, alternating right hand and leg with left hand and leg.

Points to remember
● The idea of this technique is that when one person uses force to press forward the other should turn his waist to dissolve that force. The former should not lean forward and the latter, when shifting weight back, should not lean back.
● Movements of arms and legs should not be stiff and should be coordinated throughout.

BASIC TWO-HAND TECHNIQUES

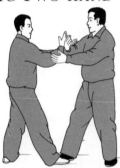
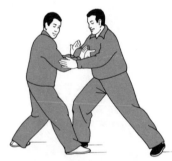
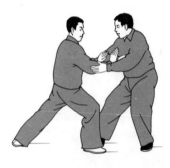

Starting position Stand facing each other. Both half turn to left and step forward with right foot. Both raise right hand, elbow bent and backs of hands lightly touching each other. Left-hand palm of each touches other's right elbow.
1–2 A turn over right hand so that palm is touching **B**'s right wrist and force **B** to withdraw his right arm toward his chest in a forward and downward move; at same time move left hand forward in same direction from **B**'s elbow.

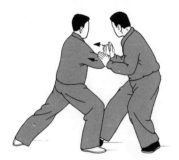
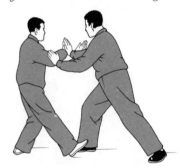
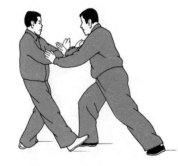

3 B accept **A**'s forward force with arm and retreat with left hand resting on **A**'s right elbow. Bend left leg slightly, shift weight backward, turn torso to right and use right arm to divert **A**'s push to right, thus dissolving **A**'s force.
4–5 B turn over right hand so that palm touches **A**'s right wrist; at same time push both palms forward and down forcing **A** to withdraw his right arm toward his chest; at same time move left hand forward in same direction from **A**'s elbow.
6 A repeat step 3 and use same technique to dissolve **B**'s force. Repeat exercise many times.

TUISHOU ON FIXED FEET

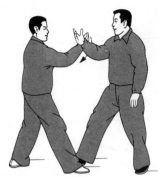

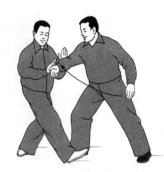

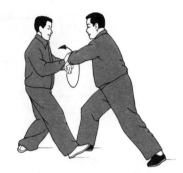

Starting position *Both half turn to left and put right foot forward. Raise right hand with elbow bent and backs of hands lightly touching each other. Do not press too hard or yield too much to each other.*

*1 **A** retreat by turning body to right and withdrawing right arm. Turn right hand over and touch **B**'s right*

*wrist; at same time gently hold **B**'s right elbow with left hand and taking advantage of **B**'s forward force bend left knee and turn waist to right, hands in a pull-back movement, inviting **B**'s arm in.*

*2–3 **B** follow **A**'s withdrawing movement, bend right knee and shift weight forward; at same time move left hand inside right forearm and*

*press it toward **A**'s chest and try to force **A** to abandon his effort. Now **A** take advantage of **B**'s forward force and bend left leg; pull chest in and turn waist to left; at same time press **B**'s right arm down and to the left with both hands, thereby neutralizing **B**'s pressing force.*

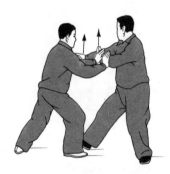

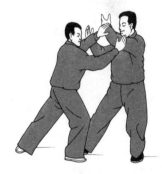

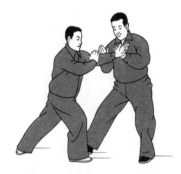

*4 **A** move right hand to **B**'s left elbow and left hand to **B**'s left wrist and push forward with palms.*

*5–6 **B** accept **A**'s push with left*

*arm and pull right hand out to stroke **A**'s left elbow; at same time bend left leg, shift weight backward and turn body slightly to left. Ward*

*off **A**'s force with left arm and divert **A**'s arm upward with both hands, and with a withdrawal movement lure **A**'s arm in.*

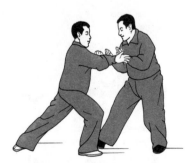

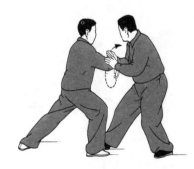

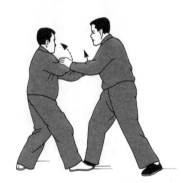

*7 **A** take immediate advantage of **B**'s move and with right hand supporting inside of left elbow press*

*firmly toward **B**'s chest.*

*8 **B** accept **A**'s forward force and bend left leg, pull chest in and move*

*hands to touch **A**'s right elbow.*

*9 Shift weight forward and push **A**'s right arm away to right.*

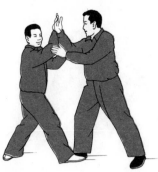

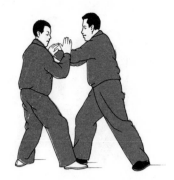

10 *A raise right hand to ward off B's push and at same time move left hand to hold B's right elbow and turn body to right.*

11 *B press right arm forward toward A's chest. A instead of resisting, hold B's left wrist with left hand and push B's left elbow*

gently with right hand; turn body to left and divert B's pressure.

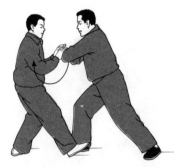

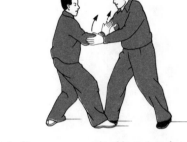

12 *B with right leg bent take advantage of situation by pressing left arm forward.*
13 *When A responds by pushing*

forward with both hands B move left hand from underneath A's hands to hold A's right elbow and shift weight backward, luring A in.

At this point A push forward. Repeat exercise many times backward and forward, without moving feet.

TUISHOU WITH FEET MOVING

ADVANCE THREE STEPS, RETREAT TWO STEPS

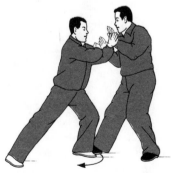

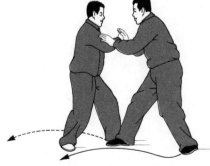

Starting position *Stand facing each other, A put left foot forward and B put right foot forward (on outside of A's left foot). Both raise left hand with elbow bent and*

backs of hands lightly touching each other. Each person's right hand should touch the other's left elbow.
1 *A press forward with left arm and rest right hand on inside of left*

elbow; B push A's arm down with both hands.
2 *B place right foot on inside of A's left foot (first advance step) and push A's arm with both hands.*▶

太极推手

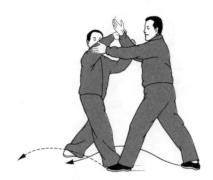

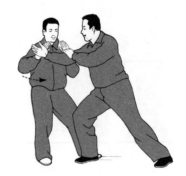

3 *A step back with left foot (first retreat step), take hold of **B's** right hand with right hand and stroke **B's** right elbow with left hand. **B** take advantage of **A's** retreat and bring left foot forward (second advance step) and land it just outside **A's** right foot and get ready to press forward with right arm.*

4 *A step back with right foot (second retreat step), at same time lead **B's** arm to right with both hands. Following **A's** retreat, **B** bring right foot forward again and place it just inside **A's** left foot (third advance step) with right knee bent and arm pressing forward.*

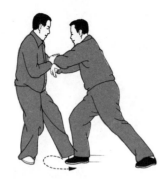

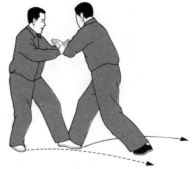

5 *A bend right knee slightly, shift weight backward and push at **B's** arms with hands.*

6 *A take advantage of **B** pressing forward and turn waist slightly to left, lift left foot and land it on inside of **B's** right foot (**A's** first advance step) and push forward with both hands.*

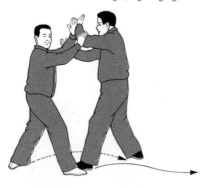

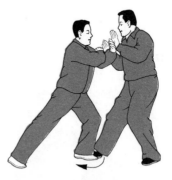

7 *B step back with right foot and at same time move right hand round and take hold of **A's** left elbow in retreat. **A** take advantage by bringing right foot forward and landing it just outside **B's** left foot (**A's** second advance step).*

8 *B retreat with left foot; **A** follow with left foot and place it just inside **B's** right foot, press forward again with left arm. **B** push **A's** arm downward with both hands and return to step 1.*

This exercise can be repeated over and over again, advancing and retreating, advancing and retreating, and so on.

ADVANCE THREE STEPS, RETREAT THREE STEPS

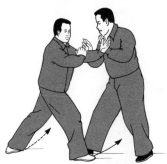
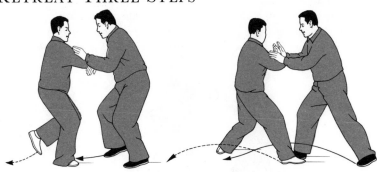

Starting position *Both half turn to left and step forward with right foot. Both raise right hand, elbow bent and backs of hands lightly touching each other; do not press or recoil from each other too much.*

1–3 *A press forward with left arm, aiming at B's chest, support inside of left elbow with right hand and bend right leg. B retreat and push at A's arm with both hands; at same time B lift right foot and*

step forward and A lift foot and step backward. B take hold of A's right hand with right hand causing A's right arm to fold and stroke A's right elbow with left hand.

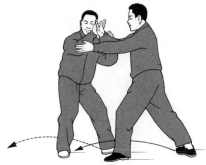
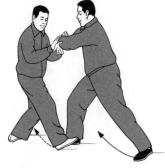

4–5 *B advance again with left foot and A retreat with right foot. A raise right hand to ward off B's push and at same time move left hand to hold B's right elbow and*

turn body to right. B continue to advance with right foot and A continue to retreat with left foot. B press forward with left arm, aiming at A's chest, support inside of left

elbow with right hand. A push at B's arm with both hands while retreating.

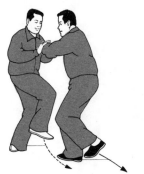
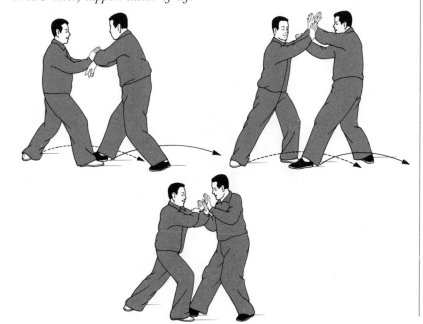

6–10 *Repeat steps 1–5, but A start by stepping forward with right foot and B start by stepping back with left foot.*

DA LU (TO PULL BACK)

This is a special technique in taiji and on the surface looks like a retreating or falling back movement but is in fact a positive and not a negative movement. It involves taking hold of one's opponent's elbow and wrist with both hands in order to pull back his hand and body, thus neutralizing his forward force. No element of conflict is involved.

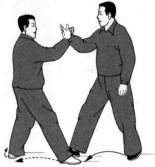

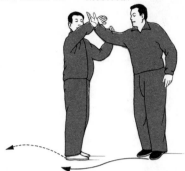

Starting position Both half turn to left and put right foot forward. Both raise right hand, elbow bent and backs of hands lightly touching each other.

1 **A** turn over right hand, hold **B's** right wrist gently and rest left hand on **B's** right elbow. At same time pivot on ball of left foot, half turn to right, bring right foot back and start the pulling back movement. **B** move left foot next to right foot and shift weight forward.

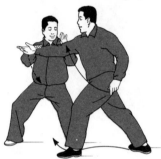

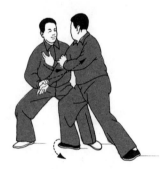

2 **A** turn body to right and step back with right foot. At same time keep pulling back **B's** arm with both hands, forcing **B** to step forward with left foot. **B** should feel slightly unbalanced due to force of **A's** pulling.

3 Following **A's** pulling, **B** bring right foot forward, land it just inside **A's** left foot and shift weight onto right leg; at same time hold inside of own right arm with left hand and lean shoulder lightly against **A's** chest.

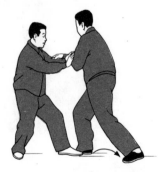

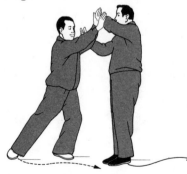

4–5 **A** take advantage of **B's** move, intercept **B's** right arm with left arm and elbow and turn body slightly to right so as to neutralize **B's** forward force. **A** then pull chest in, turn waist to left and shift weight to right leg; at same time start to push forward instead of pulling back by putting left hand on **B's** left hand and right hand on **B's** left elbow and bring left foot forward so that it lands on inside of **B's** right foot.

6 **B** accept **A's** onward push and ward off **A's** hands with left forearm and move right arm around to hold **A's** left elbow; at same time **B** pull right foot back, turn body slightly to left and start to pull. As **B** moves, **A** bend left leg and shift weight forward.

太极推手

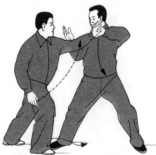

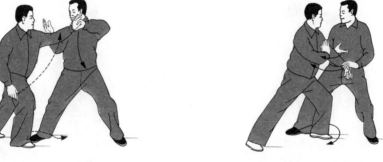

7 **B** *turn body to left, step back with left foot, knee bent; at same time continue the pulling movement: hold* **A's** *left wrist with left hand and left elbow with right hand.* **A**

follow by taking a large step forward with right foot and shifting weight onto right leg.
8 **A** *follow with left foot, land it on inside of* **B's** *right foot and shift*

weight forward. At same time, with right hand pressing inside of left arm, lean shoulder toward **B's** *chest.*

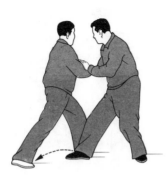

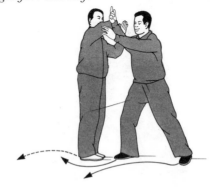

The above steps show that **A** *and* **B** *both advance and retreat once and thus complete a cycle. If* **B** *advances*

with right foot and pushes forward while **A** *retreats with left foot and pulls back, this exercise can easily*

be repeated over and over again in continuous cycles.

CHANGING-HANDS METHOD

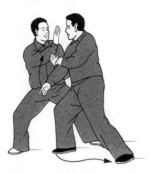

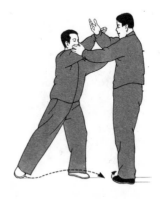

1 **B** *step forward with left foot and lean right arm and shoulder against* **A's** *chest; take another step forward with right foot and* **A** *step back with right foot.* **A***, while stepping back, turn body to right*

and receive and neutralize **B's** *forward force with left arm and at same time quickly raise right hand as though about to slap* **B's** *face.*
2 **B** *raise right arm to ward off* **A's** *hand and step back with right*

foot. At same time turn body to right, keeping feet together, and pull **A** *to right by holding* **A's** *right wrist with right hand and right elbow with left hand.* ▶

太极推手

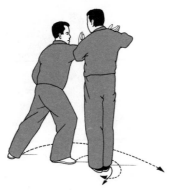
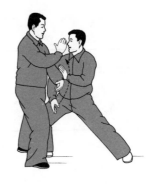

3 *A* *follow with right foot, shift weight forward and turn to left.*
4 *B* *keep turning to right, step back with right foot and continue pulling* *movement.* *A* *drawn by* *B's* *pulling power, step forward with left foot, make a complete right turn and land right foot on inside of* *B's* *left foot;* *at same time push inside of right arm with left hand and lean forward against* *B's* *chest.*

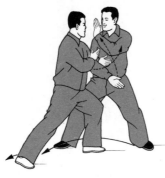
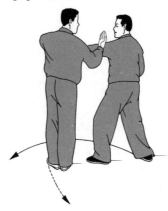

Steps 5–8 are the opposite of steps 1–4 using the left arm instead of the right. Basic movements involving advances and retreats are the same.

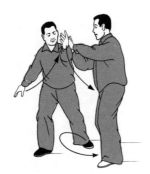
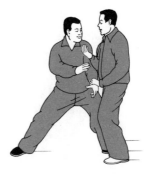

5–8 *A* *step forward and lean left arm and shoulder against* *B's* *chest.* *B* *turn body to left, using right arm to receive and neutralize* *A's* *onward force. At same time raise left hand quickly as though about to slap* *A's* *face.* *A* *use left hand to pull* *B's* *left arm off to left.* *B* *follow with left arm and press it against* *A's* *chest.*
This exercise can be repeated over and over again in cycles.

EXERCISES TO PREVENT CERTAIN DISEASES

PRINCIPLES

All exercises, if done properly, are good for health and this section contains some traditional Chinese exercises that are especially designed to prevent certain diseases. They have been revised by modern experts. A section describing types of baths that are of therapeutic value is also included.

The physical effects of these exercises are specifically named. The 18 therapies really belong in the external forms of exercise, but since they are explicitly described in the Chinese text as having a curative effect on joint diseases and certain other internal disorders they are included here.

The 36 movements of the 18 therapies cover every part of the body and touch upon every joint. The variety of movements and positions is great, and since the exercises are divided into sets and broken down into movements they are easy to learn. Rhythm is important and the exercises should be done slowly. It is also helpful to count the beats as you go along. Postures and positions must be followed accurately; body and limbs should be stretched as much as possible and breathing should be harmonious with other body movements.

Breathing exercises, or qigong as they are called in China, are also a form of internal exercise. Learners who expect to be able to perform extraordinary feats like resisting bullets or heavy objects after having mastered qigong will be disappointed. In this book qigong is purely therapeutic and puts emphasis on mind control to achieve complete relaxation. Beginners are advised not to practice qigong when tired since they may fall asleep.

The eye exercises are simple to learn and fun to do. They have instant results and one's eyes feel immediately rested. An important thing to remember when doing these exercises is that one must pinpoint the acupuncture points around the eyes accurately and it is therefore important to study the illustrations carefully.

Moving on to self-massage, learn by heart the ten different ways of using your hands and fingers before embarking on the exercise. A list of ten Chinese terms and their meanings is included. It is difficult to describe each term exactly in English, but hopefully the illustrations will give a clearer idea. A complicated and detailed description of the 300–400 acupuncture points all over the body is omitted here since that knowledge is not required for the self-massage methods in this book.

The therapeutic value of baths is well known. The techniques described in this book are commonly practiced in China and can easily be adapted to Western society.

練功十八法
THE 18 THERAPIES

The 18 therapies actually involve 36 movements. The first three sets of exercises with 18 movements are designed to relieve or prevent pains in the neck, shoulders, waist and legs. The second three sets of exercises which also have 18 movements are ideal for sufferers of arthritis and internal disorders.

These exercises should be done slowly and in a continuous flow. Each has eight steps and when exercising it is often helpful to count the beats "one . . . two . . . three . . . four" in rhythm.

THE FIRST SET

This set of exercises relieves pain in neck and shoulders.

STRENGTHENING THE NECK

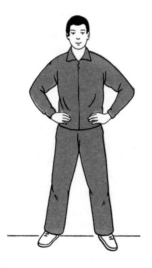 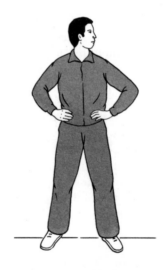

Preparation *Stand with feet apart at a distance slightly wider than shoulder width. Rest hands gently on waist.*
1 Turn head to left as far as possible, following movement with eyes.
2 Return to preparation position.
3 Turn head to right as far as possible, following movement with eyes.

4 Return to preparation position.
5 Bend head back to look at sky.
6 Return to preparation position.
7 Bend head forward to look at ground.
8 Return to preparation position. Repeat exercise two to four times, each time to a count of eight.

Points to remember
● *When turning and bending head keep body straight.*
● *When bending head forward touch breastbone with chin.*

Affected areas Muscles in neck.

Physical effects Relieves tension and pain in neck and cures a stiff neck.

STRENGTHENING THE SHOULDERS

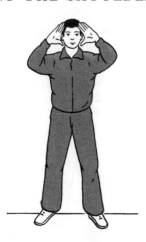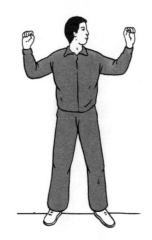

练功十八法

Preparation *Stand with feet apart at a distance slightly wider than shoulder width. Circle head with open palms and look straight ahead.*
1 Move hands to side and expand chest. At same time clench fists loosely and turn head to left. Keeping elbows down, look through fists, which should be hollow.

2 Return to preparation position.
3–4 Repeat steps 1–2, but in opposite direction.
Repeat exercise two to four times, each time to a count of eight.

Points to remember
- *When expanding chest keep shoulders back.*
- *Keep elbows level.*

Affected areas Muscles in neck, shoulders, back and upper arms.

Physical effects Relieves tension and stiffness in neck, shoulders and back and also numbness in arms. Relaxes chest area.

EXTENDING THE HANDS

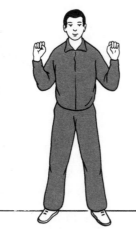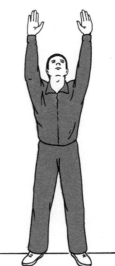

Preparation *Stand with feet apart at a distance slightly wider than shoulder width. Clench fists loosely and hold them up as though holding a bar in front of you.*
1 Raise arms above head and unclench fists with palms facing out. Bend head back and look at thumbs.

2 Return to preparation position.
Repeat exercise two to four times, each time to a count of eight.

Points to remember
- *When raising arms expand chest and contract abdomen. Do not hold breath.*

Affected areas Muscles in neck and around waist.

Physical effects Relieves tension and stiffness in neck, shoulders, back and waist. Good for shoulder joints.

EXPANDING THE CHEST

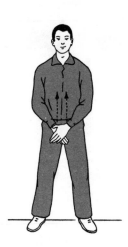
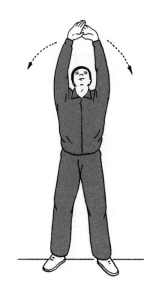

Preparation *Stand with feet apart at a distance slightly wider than shoulder width and cross hands in front of abdomen.*
1 With hands still crossed raise arms and keep eyes on hands.
2 Drop arms to side and return to preparation position.

Repeat exercise two to four times, each time to a count of eight.

Points to remember
● *When raising arms keep head up, chest out and abdomen contracted.*

Affected areas Neck, shoulders and waist.

Physical effects Strengthens shoulder joints, neck and back.

FLAPPING WINGS

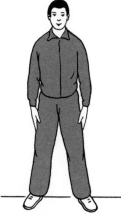
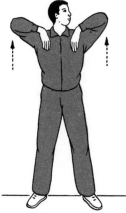
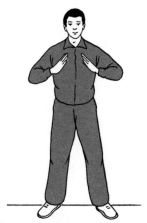

Preparation *Stand with feet apart at a distance slightly wider than shoulder width.*
1 Bend arms and raise elbows high above shoulders, drop hands with backs of hands facing each other. At same time turn head to left.

2 Drop elbows, lift hands up and push down slowly; return to preparation position.
3–4 Repeat steps 1–2, but in opposite direction.
Repeat exercise two to four times, each time to a count of eight.

Points to remember
● *When raising elbows do not shrug shoulders.*
● *Relax wrists throughout exercise.*

Affected areas Shoulders and chest.

Physical effects Strengthens shoulder joints and upper arms.

RAISING ONE ARM

Preparation *Stand with feet apart at a distance slightly wider than shoulder width.*
1 Raise left arm, palm up, keeping eyes on back of hand. At same time bend right arm and hold hand behind back.
2 Return to preparation position, keeping eyes on left hand.
3–4 Repeat steps 1–2, but raise right arm and put left arm behind back.
Repeat exercise two to four times, each time to a count of eight.

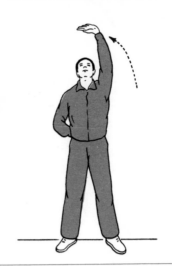

Points to remember
● *When raising arm keep it straight and follow hand with eyes.*

Affected areas When raising arm and turning up palm, muscles in neck and shoulder are affected.

Physical effects Strengthens shoulder joints and relieves pain in neck, shoulders and waist.

THE SECOND SET

This set of exercises relieves pain and stiffness in the waist.

STRETCHING WITH HANDS UP

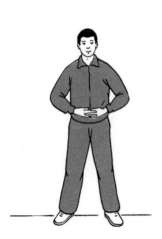
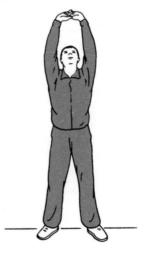
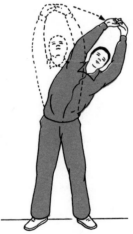

Preparation *Stand with feet apart at a distance slightly wider than shoulder width. Place hands against abdomen, fingers interlocked and palms up.*
1 Lift hands above head, turn palms right over and, with head bent back and chest out, push up.
2 Stretch arms and bend to left.

3 Repeat step 2.
4 Bring arms down to side and return to preparation position.
5–8 Repeat steps 1–4, but in opposite direction.
Repeat exercise two to four times, each time to a count of eight.

Points to remember
● *When pushing up keep elbows and body straight.*

Affected areas Neck and waist and also shoulders, arms and fingers.

Physical effects Strengthens neck and shoulder joints and waist and keeps vertebral column straight.

練功十八法

PUSHING AWAY WHILE TWISTING

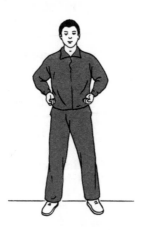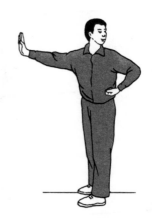

Preparation *Stand with feet apart at a distance slightly wider than shoulder width, fists at waist.*
1 Open right fist and push forward, while twisting body to left until left elbow and right arm are in line with each other. Keep eyes on left elbow.

2 Return to preparation position.
3–4 Repeat steps 1–2, but in opposite direction.
Repeat exercise two to four times, each time to a count of eight.

Points to remember
● *While turning body keep feet still and legs straight.*

Affected areas Waist, shoulders, neck and back.

Physical effects Relieves stiffness in neck, waist and shoulders.

ROTATING THE PELVIS

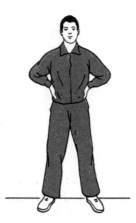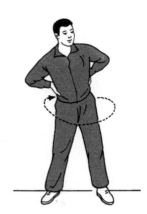

Preparation *Stand with feet apart at a distance slightly wider than shoulder width, hands at waist, thumbs in front.*
1 Rotate pelvis clockwise to a count of four: "one, two, three, four."

2 Rotate pelvis counterclockwise to a count of four: "five, six, seven, eight."

Points to remember
● *When rotating pelvis start with a small circle and gradually expand it.*
● *Keep legs straight and feet still.*
● *Use hands to support body.*

Affected area Waist.

Physical effects Relieves stiffness in waist and sacrum.

ARMS AND WAIST

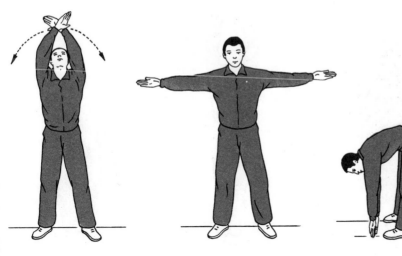

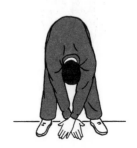

Preparation *Stand with feet apart at a distance slightly wider than shoulder width and cross hands in front of abdomen.*
1 Lift arms above head. Bend head back, keep eyes on backs of hands, chest out and abdomen contracted.
2 Lower arms to shoulder level, palms up.

3 Turn palms over and bend forward to touch ground with fingers.
4 Cross hands.
5–8 Repeat steps 1–4 and return to preparation position.
Repeat exercise two to four times to a count of eight.

Points to remember
● *Keep legs straight.*

Affected areas Waist and legs.

Physical effects Relieves pain and stiffness in neck, back and waist.

THRUSTING THE HAND WITH ONE LEG BENT, ONE LEG STRAIGHT

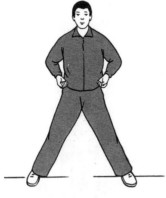

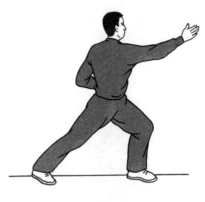

Preparation *Stand with legs wide apart, fists at waist.*
1 Turn to left and, keeping right leg straight, bend left knee. At same time open right fist and thrust hand forward.
2 Return to preparation position.

3–4 Repeat steps 1–2, but in opposite direction.
Repeat exercise two to four times, each time to a count of eight.

Points to remember
● *When doing step 1 keep arm, waist and leg straight.*

Affected areas Waist and legs.

Physical effects Relieves stiffness and numbness in neck, waist, back, arms and legs.

TOUCHING THE FEET WITH HANDS

練功十八法

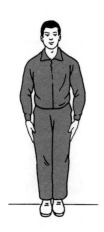
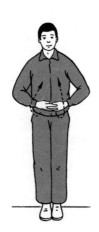
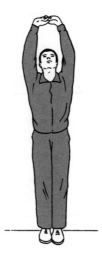
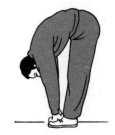

Preparation *Stand to attention.*
1 Place hands in front of abdomen with fingers interlocked and palms facing up.
2 Lift hands with palms up until arms are straight.
3 Bend forward until both hands touch feet.

4 Return to preparation position. Repeat exercise two to four times, each time to a count of eight.

Points to remember
● *When bending forward keep knees straight and stretch arms as far as possible.*

Affected areas When stretching, neck and waist. When bending, waist and legs.

Physical effects Relieves stiffness in waist, back and legs.

THE THIRD SET

This set prevents and relieves pain in hips and legs.

ROTATING THE KNEES

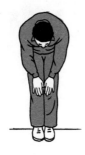
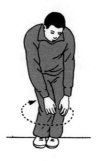

Preparation *Bend forward and place hands on knees.*
1 Rotate knees clockwise.
2 Return to preparation position. Repeat exercise two to four times, each time to a count of eight. Do

first eight movements clockwise and second eight counterclockwise.

Points to remember
● *When rotating knees make circle as large as possible.*

Affected areas Knees and ankles.

Physical effects Relieves stiffness and prevents weakness in knees and ankles.

練功十八法

THE 45-DEGREE TURN

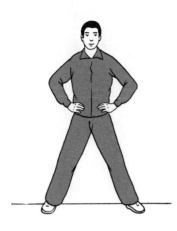 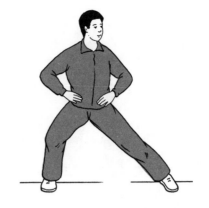

Preparation *Stand with legs wide apart, hands holding waist with thumbs behind you.*
1 Bend right knee and turn body to left at a 45-degree angle.
2 Return to preparation position.
3 Bend left knee and turn body to right at a 45-degree angle.

4 Repeat step 2.
Repeat exercise two to four times, each time to a count of eight.

Points to remember
● *When bending knee keep it in a vertical line with foot. The body must also be straight.*

Affected areas Thigh and leg muscles.

Physical effects Relieves stiffness in waist, hips, legs, knees and also ankles.

SQUATTING

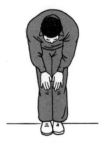 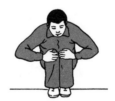 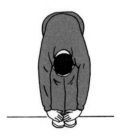

Preparation *Stand to attention.*
1 Bend forward, place hands on knees and keep legs straight.
2 Squat with hands on knees.
3 Place hands on top of feet and straighten legs.
4 Return to preparation position.

Repeat exercise two to four times, each time to a count of eight.

Points to remember
● *When bending forward keep knee joints straight and stretch arms as far as possible.*

Affected areas When squatting, thighs and knees. When straightening up, thighs and legs.

Physical effects Relieves stiffness in hips, knees and legs.

BENDING AND STRETCHING

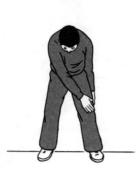

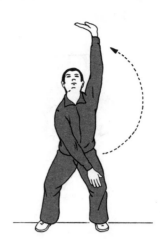

Preparation *Stand with legs shoulder-width apart.*
1 Bend forward, place right hand on left knee; keep legs straight.
2 Bend knees slightly, lift left hand above head, palm up, and keep eyes on back of hand.
3 Straighten legs and place left hand on right knee.
4 Return to preparation position.

5–8 Repeat steps 1–4, but in opposite direction.
Repeat exercise two to four times, each time to a count of eight.

Points to remember
● *This exercise may be done again and again without a break by repeating step 2, but in opposite direction after step 3.*

● *When bending knees do not move feet and keep upper body straight.*

Affected areas Neck, shoulder, waist and leg muscles.

Physical effects Relieves pain and stiffness in neck, shoulder, waist and legs.

CLASPING THE KNEE TOWARD CHEST

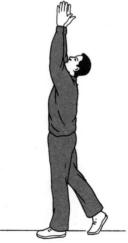

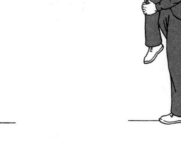

Preparation *Stand to attention.*
1 Step forward with left foot and, keeping right heel off ground, shift weight to left leg. At same time lift arms above head with palms facing each other; keep head back and chest high.
2 Raise right knee and drop arms to side. Clasp knee tightly toward chest and keep left leg straight.

3 Repeat step 1.
4 Return to preparation position.
5–8 Repeat steps 1–4, but in opposite direction.
Repeat exercise two to four times, each time to a count of eight.

Points to remember
● *When clasping knee toward chest keep supporting leg straight and steady.*

Affected areas Legs and knees.

Physical effects Relieves stiffness in hips and legs; increases flexibility of knees.

THE HERO'S STROLL

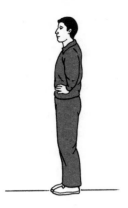 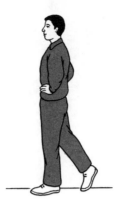 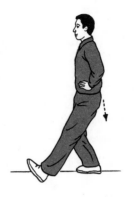

Preparation *Stand straight, hands at waist.*
1 Step forward with left foot, heel first. Shift weight to left leg and lift right heel off ground.
2 Lower right heel, bend right knee slightly and shift weight to right leg. Lift left foot so that only heel is touching ground.
3–4 Repeat steps 1–2, but change legs round.
5 Shift weight to right leg and lift left heel off ground.

6 Shift weight back to left leg, bend left knee and lift right foot so that only heel is touching ground.
7 Straighten left leg, step back with right foot and bend right knee slightly. Shift weight to right leg.
8 Return to preparation position. Repeat exercise two to four times, each time to a count of eight.

Points to remember
● *Keep upper body straight throughout exercise.*

● *When stepping forward and back keep head high and chest out.*

Affected areas When weight is on left leg, muscles in left leg and right ankle are felt. When weight is on right leg, muscles in right leg and left ankle are felt.

Physical effects Relieves stiffness in legs and knees and limbers up knee and ankle joints.

THE FOURTH SET

This set relieves and prevents pain in leg and arm joints.

HORSE RIDING
Preparation *Stand with feet apart at a distance slightly wider than shoulder width, fists at waist.*
1 Bend knees and assume a horse-riding position. At same time turn arms in, open fists and thrust open palms forward with middle fingers touching each other.
2 Return to preparation position. Repeat exercise two to four times, each time to a count of eight.

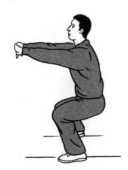

Points to remember
● *When thrusting palms forward turn wrists in and keep arms as straight as possible.*

Affected areas Wrist and thighs.

Physical effects Relieves stiffness in arms and legs and especially knees.

練功十八法

SQUATTING WITH CROSSED LEGS

Preparation *Stand with feet apart at a distance slightly wider than shoulder width, fists at waist.*
1 Twist body to left, cross right leg over left leg and squat. At same time push left palm out to left and turn head to right.
2 Return to preparation position.
3–4 Repeat steps 1–2, but in opposite direction.

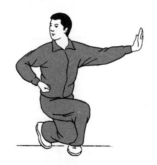

Repeat exercise two to four times, each time to a count of eight.

Points to remember
● *When squatting keep body straight and steady.*

Affected areas Legs and arms.

Physical effects Relieves stiffness in neck, back and all joints.

SEARCHING – UP AND DOWN, LEFT AND RIGHT

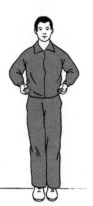 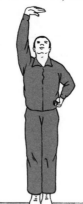 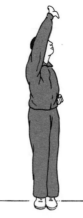 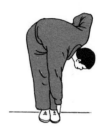

Preparation *Stand straight, fists at waist, palms up.*
1 Unclench right fist and lift above head, eyes following back of hand.
2 Twist body to left at a 90-degree angle.
3 Bring right hand down along left side and bend forward to touch outside of left foot.
4 Twist body to right while

passing right palm over top of both feet and side of right leg; return to preparation position.
5–8 Repeat steps 1–4, but in opposite direction.
Repeat exercise two to four times, each time to a count of eight.

Points to remember
● *When bending forward keep knees straight.*

Affected areas Shoulders, arms, waist and legs.

Physical effects Relieves pain and stiffness in neck, shoulders, waist and legs.

TWISTING THE BODY AND LOOKING BACKWARD

Preparation *Stand with legs wide apart, fists at waist.*
1 Twist body to left and with right leg straight and left leg bent, look over left shoulder. At same time stretch right arm up, palm facing out; keep right arm and leg in straight line.
2 Return to preparation position.
3–4 Repeat steps 1–2, but in opposite direction.
Repeat exercise two to four times, each time to a count of eight.

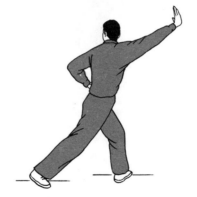

Points to remember
● *When doing steps 1 and 3 keep right leg straight and heel on ground.*

Affected areas Neck, shoulders, waist and legs.

Physical effects Relieves pain and stiffness in neck, shoulders, waist and legs.

STRETCHING THE LEGS

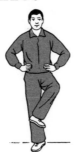
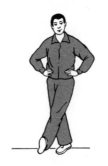

Preparation *Stand with legs shoulder-width apart and hands at waist, thumbs pointing back.*
1 Lift left leg and twist heel toward right and stretch leg firmly.
2 Return to preparation position.
3 Repeat step 1, but with right leg.

4 Return to preparation position. Repeat exercise two to four times, each time to a count of eight.

Points to remember
● *Keep upper body firm and use heel to exert force.*

Affected areas Legs.

Physical effects Relieves pain and stiffness in thighs and knee joints.

KICKING THE SHUTTLECOCK

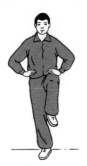
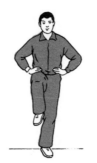
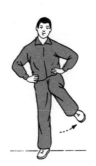
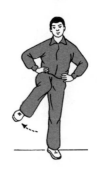

Preparation *Stand straight, hands at waist, thumbs pointing back.*

1 Lift left leg and kick up.
2 Lift right leg and kick up.
3 Lift left knee and kick sideways.

4 Lift right knee and kick sideways.

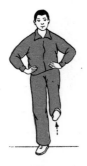
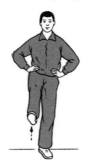
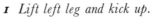
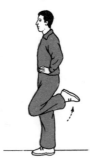
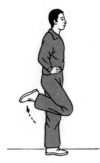

5 Lift left leg and kick forward.
6 Lift right leg and kick forward.
7 Bend left leg and kick back.
8 Bend right leg and kick back.
Return to preparation position after each step.
Repeat exercise two to four times, each time to a count of eight.

Points to remember
● *Keep leg that is not kicking straight and steady.*
● *When kicking back with heel use enough force so that heel is so high that it causes thigh to be vertical with ground.*

Affected areas Thighs and legs.

Physical effects Relieves pain and stiffness in hip bones and joints.

THE FIFTH SET

This set prevents and relieves tennis elbow and strained tendons.

PUSHING AWAY

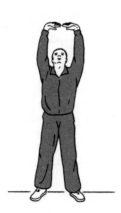
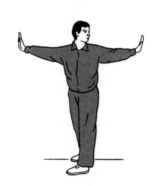
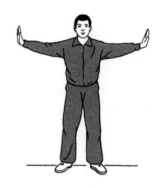

Preparation *Stand with feet apart at a distance slightly wider than shoulder width with fists at waist.*
1 Unclench fists and with palms up and middle fingers pointing at each other, stretch arms up toward sky; keep eyes on back of hands.
2 Return to preparation position.
3 Unclench fists and stretch arms to the sides, palms facing out. At same

time twist body to left, keeping eyes on back of left hand.
4 Repeat step 2.
5 Repeat step 3, but in opposite direction.
6 Repeat step 2.
7 Unclench fists, stretch arms to sides, palms facing out, and look ahead.
8 Return to preparation position.
Repeat exercise two to four times, each time to a count of eight.

Points to remember
● *When twisting body keep it straight and do not move feet.*

Affected areas Neck, shoulders, elbows, wrists and fingers.

Physical effects Relieves tennis elbow and stiffness in fingers, wrists, neck, shoulders and waist.

ARCHERY

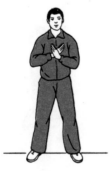
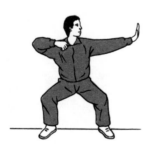
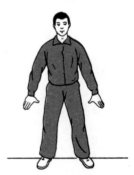

Preparation *Stand to attention.*
1 Step to left and cross hands in front of chest.
2 Bend knees to assume a horse-riding position. At same time stretch left arm, palm out to left, and pull right elbow to right, fist facing ground. Keep eyes on back of left hand.

3 Straighten legs and press both hands down.
4 Return to preparation position.
5–8 Repeat steps 1–4, but in opposite direction.
Repeat exercise two to four times, each time to a count of eight.

Points to remember
● *When doing steps 2 and 3 expand chest and keep shoulders back.*

Affected areas Forearms, wrists and fingers.

Physical effects Relieves tennis elbow and stiff fingers.

STRETCHING ARMS AND TURNING WRISTS

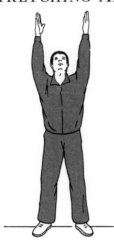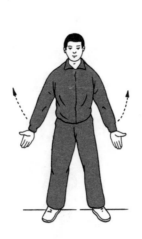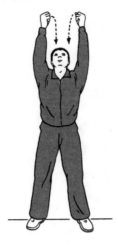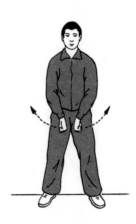

練功十八法

Preparation *Stand with feet apart at a distance slightly wider than shoulder width, fists at waist.*
1 Unclench fists and stretch arms up, palms facing each other and eyes looking up.
2 Clench fists and turn wrists out; lower arms to sides and return to preparation position. Repeat these two steps once or twice, each time to a count of eight.
3 Unclench fists and stretch arms down, palms facing out; lift arms above head, palms facing each other and eyes looking up.
4 Clench fists, turn wrists so that fists are back to back and bend elbows to bring down fists to just below waist level.
5 Return to preparation position. Repeat exercise, two steps at a time, two to four times, each time to a count of eight.

Points to remember
● *When lifting arms up expand chest.*

Affected areas Wrists, elbows, shoulders and arms.

Physical effects Relieves tennis elbow and pain in wrists, fingers and shoulders.

STRETCHING ARMS FORWARD AND BACKWARD

Preparation *Stand with feet apart at a distance slightly wider than shoulder width, fists at waist.*
1 Unclench right fist and thrust hand up with thumb extended. At the same time stretch left fist back and turn head to look at fist.
2 Return to preparation position.
3 Repeat step 1, but change hands over.
4 Return to preparation position. Repeat exercise two to four times, each time to a count of eight.

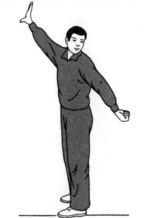

Points to remember
● *When doing step 1 form arms into straight line with shoulders extended.*

Affected areas Shoulders, arms, elbows, fingers and chest.

Physical effects Relieves tennis elbow and pain in wrists, fingers, shoulders, waist and back.

練功十八法

PUNCHING IN A HORSE-RIDING POSITION

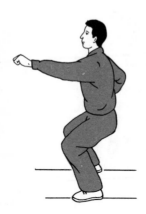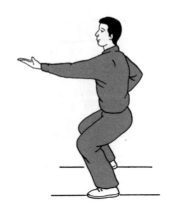

Preparation *Stand with feet apart at a distance slightly wider than shoulder width, fists at waist.*
1 Bend knees to assume a horse-riding position. At same time thrust left fist forward, palm down.
2 Unclench fist, turn palm up and return to preparation position.

3–4 Repeat steps 1–2, but with right fist.
Repeat exercise two to four times, each time to a count of eight.

Points to remember
● *Keep chest expanded throughout exercise.*
● *Thrust fists forward.*

Affected areas Arms, wrists, fingers and legs.

Physical effects Relieves tennis elbow and pain in wrists, fingers, neck, shoulders and waist.

TWISTING THE BODY TO LEFT AND RIGHT

Preparation *Stand straight with feet apart at a distance slightly wider than shoulder width.*
1 Turn upper body to left, open right hand and push left shoulder with thumb down; place back of left hand against back of waist and look over left shoulder.
2 Return to preparation position.
3–4 Repeat steps 1–2, but in opposite direction.
Repeat exercise two to four times, each time to a count of eight.

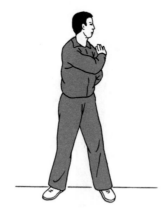

Points to remember
● *When pushing shoulder with open hand do not raise elbow and keep feet still.*
● *Do whole exercise slowly and twist body as far as possible.*

Affected areas Neck, shoulders, elbows and wrists.

Physical effects Relieves tennis elbow and pain in shoulders, back and waist.

THE SIXTH SET

This set prevents and cures disorders of internal organs.

練功十八法

RUBBING THE FACE

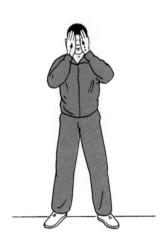
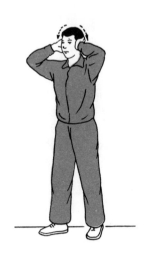
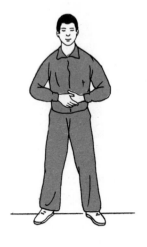

Preparation *Stand straight with feet shoulder-width apart.*
1 Using middle fingers, massage face, starting from corners of mouth and moving up to forehead; then use whole hands and rub face with a circular movement 8–16 times.
2 Rub face by moving palms upward until they reach hair on temples, then move palms down back of head, behind ears to face. Repeat movement 8–16 times.

3 Place hand against upper abdomen, look straight ahead and lick palate with tongue. With right thumb rub between thumb and index finger of left hand 24–36 times. Change hands and repeat movement 24–36 times.

Points to remember
● *When massaging face and head use pressure.*
● *When rubbing hand with thumb close eyes and concentrate.*

Affected areas Face and area between thumb and index finger.

Physical effects Relieves insomnia, nervousness, palpitations, dizziness and stomach disorders.

MASSAGING CHEST AND ABDOMEN

Preparation *Stand with feet apart at a distance slightly wider than shoulder width. Place right hand against upper abdomen and left hand on top of right hand.*
1 Massage upper abdomen eight times with small circular movements. Massage area from lower abdomen to chest eight times with large circular movements.
2 Massage same areas, but in opposite direction, first with large then with small circular movements.

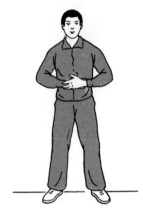

Points to remember
● *Relax and press hands tightly against abdomen.*
● *Look straight ahead.*

Affected areas Massage brings warmth to abdomen and tends to cause wind, which brings relaxation and comfort to stomach.

Physical effects Corrects disorders in stomach and intestines and also relieves pain in waist and back.

COMBING SCALP

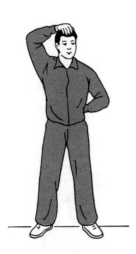 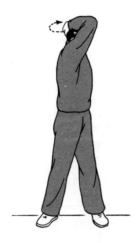 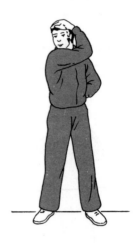

Preparation *Stand straight with feet apart at a distance slightly wider than shoulder width.*
1 *Hold top of head firmly with right hand, four fingers in front; place back of left hand against lower back.*
2 *Twist body toward left and run fingers through hair to neck bone.*
3 *Move right palm up against*

right side of head, passing right ear, until it reaches left side of forehead. At same time twist head and body to right.
4 *Return to preparation position.*
5–8 *Repeat steps 1–4, but in opposite direction.*
Repeat exercise two to four times, each time to a count of eight.

Points to remember
● *Press whole hand firmly against head.*
● *Do exercise slowly and in a continuous flow.*

Affected areas Head and waist.

Physical effects Alleviates dizziness, blurred vision, insomnia and palpitations.

LIFTING THE KNEE

Preparation *Stand to attention, fists at waist, palms up.*
1 *Shift weight to left foot and lift right knee. At same time unclench fists and press right hand down and lift left hand up, palm up, keeping eyes on back of hand.*
2 *Return to preparation position.*
3–4 *Repeat steps 1–2, but in opposite direction.*
Repeat exercise two to four times, each time to a count of eight.

Points to remember
● *When lifting knee keep body straight and stretch arms as far as possible.*

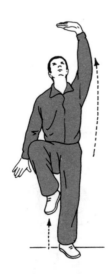

Affected areas Neck, shoulders, arms, back, waist and legs.

Physical effects Good for weak spleen, stomach and also indigestion.

BENDING AND TWISTING

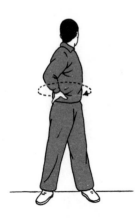 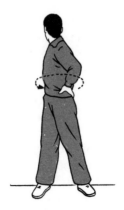 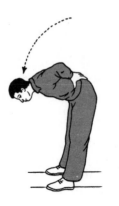 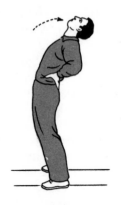

練功十八法

Preparation Stand with feet apart at a distance slightly wider than shoulder width, fists at waist.
1 Unclench fists and with palms up and middle fingers pointing at each other stretch arms up toward sky; keep eyes on backs of hands.
2 Lower arms and place hands at waist, thumbs in front.
3 Twist body toward left and back, eyes following movement.

4 Twist body toward right and back, eyes following movement.
5 Return to position in step 2.
6 Bend forward.
7 Bend back.
8 Return to preparation position. Repeat exercise two to four times, each time to a count of eight.

Points to remember
● *When twisting body keep both feet still.*
● *When bending forward and back, keep knees straight.*

Affected areas Neck, shoulders and waist.

Physical effects Good for kidney deficiency and relieves pain in back and waist.

STRETCHING ARMS AND EXPANDING CHEST

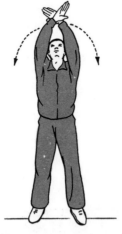 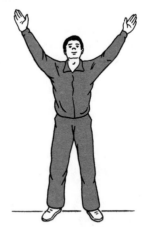

Preparation Stand straight with feet slightly apart.
1 In one movement raise arms crosswise above head, bend head back, look up, lift heels and breathe in deeply.

2 In one motion uncross arms and lower them, lower heels, breathe out and return to preparation position.

Points to remember
● *Breath naturally throughout.*
● *When raising arms stretch upper arms.*

Affected areas Chest, neck and shoulders.

Physical effects Helps prevent disease in respiratory and digestive systems.

气功

BREATHING

Breathing exercises, otherwise known as qigong, are uniquely Chinese and traditionally used as a form of preventive medicine. Qi literally means air or vitality and gong means skill or strength. It is believed in ancient Chinese medicine that breathing exercises can skilfully combine the air man inhales and his inner vitality into a vital force that can cure diseases and improve his health.

There are three main aspects of qigong all of which are equally important: body posture, breathing and mind control. They must all be mastered in order to achieve good health and to prevent and cure diseases.

Qigong is especially useful in curing chronic diseases such as neurasthenia, high blood pressure, stomach ulcers, prolapse of the stomach, duodenal ulcers and constipation. The following three reasons may explain why.

1 Qigong speeds the recuperation of one's constitution; its slow breathing method induces one's psychologically agitated state to return to a more controllable condition and this is perhaps why qigong is so beneficial to sufferers of neurasthenia, high blood pressure and stomach ulcers.

2 Qigong helps one to store energy and is therefore beneficial to sufferers of chronic diseases and those who are physically weak.

3 Qigong's abdominal breathing method massages abdominal organs and this type of rhythmic massage activates the stomach and intestines and therefore enhances the digestive system. It therefore helps to cure prolapse of the stomach and constipation.

The following rules must be adhered to in order to master qigong.

1 Relax body and mind, keep posture in a natural state and do not wear tight clothes. Relax all muscles especially in the lower abdomen area and concentrate. Keep your mind free of worry and try not to let noises or lights bother you.

2 Try to control your mind and regulate your breathing by concentrating on the rhythm, length, volume and speed of each breath. Try and reach a quiet mental state, and when regulating breathing you must be aware of the meaning of the following seven words: fine, deep, long, slow, steady, unhurried and even.

3 Supplement qigong with other physical exercise so as to attain the fullest possible benefit from this physically inactive breathing exercise.

4 Proceed in an orderly way, step by step, and be patient. Start with the easy movements and gradually move on to the more difficult. Enter the quiet state slowly and at the beginning spend only 15–20 minutes on these exercises. The time can be lengthened later.

5 Spend about 10–15 minutes preparing yourself before doing qigong – stop reading or any other mental activity, and relieve yourself. Make sure that you are neither hungry nor full and avoid qigong if you have a fever, diarrhea, a cold or are in any way overtired.

The three most popular qigong methods in China today are fangsong gong (relaxation), qiangzhuang gong (strength) and neiyang gong (inner growth).

FANGSONG GONG
(RELAXATION)

Posture *Lie down on back with a large, soft pillow under head and shoulders. Relax arms and legs, close eyes lightly and close mouth with upper and lower teeth touching each other and tip of tongue resting behind upper teeth.*

Breathing *Breathe through nose finely, evenly and steadily.*

Mind control *In order to enter the quiet state, think of the word quiet when breathing in and think of*

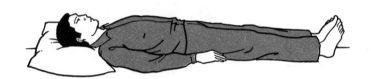

the word relax when breathing out. As you breathe out consciously relax a part of your body – head, arms, hands, chest, abdomen, back, waist, hips, legs and finally feet. After you have relaxed every part of your body start to think about relaxing your veins, nerves and internal organs.

Frequency and duration *If convalescing at home or in hospital do fangsong gong three or four times a day for about 30 minutes. If working part-time while convalescing practice it at least once or twice a day.*

Points to remember
● *You must practice for at least two or three months before you can expect to see any results.*

Physical effects Good for sufferers of chronic diseases.

气功

QIANGZHUANG GONG (STRENGTH)

This exercise can be done sitting upright, sitting cross-legged or standing.

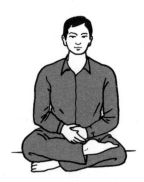

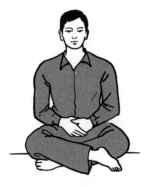

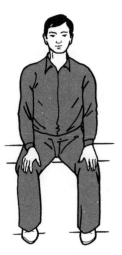

Sitting cross-legged *Sit cross-legged on a cushion in a natural manner. Keep your back straight, shoulders relaxed and head upright with chin in. Hold your hands*

together, one above the other, with thumbs crossed and palms up; keep eyes and mouth lightly closed and rest tip of tongue behind upper teeth.

Sitting upright *Sit upright on a flat stool with feet firmly on the ground. Keep legs separate, but parallel and shoulder-width apart; keep torso upright, hands on thighs, elbows naturally bent, head and spine straight, chin in, shoulders relaxed, eyes and mouth lightly closed and tip of tongue resting behind upper teeth.*

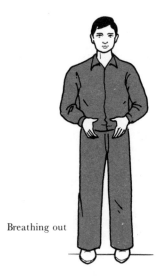

Breathing out

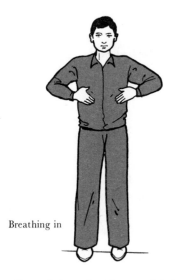

Breathing in

Standing *Stand with feet shoulder-width apart, turn toes slightly in and keep knees slightly bent. Keep back straight, arms raised, hands at shoulder level with*

elbows below shoulders, and hold arms as though embracing a large tree; keep fingers slightly bent as though holding a ball. ▶

Breathing *Breathe naturally through nose and make sure that when you breathe in and out you do it quietly, evenly and steadily. You can also practice abdominal breathing by expanding abdomen when breathing in and contracting abdomen when breathing out. Breathing should gradually become longer and deeper until you are only breathing six to eight times a minute.*

Mind control *Concentrate on lower abdomen area by using either the counting or the natural method.*

For the counting method, count your breaths – one for each inhalation and one for each exhalation. Count to ten and then repeat. As soon as distracting thoughts arise return to one and start to count again. For natural method let your concentration ride on the waves of your breathing and try and keep out distracting thoughts. Once you have gained concentration, concentrate on the lower abdomen area, which is about $1\frac{1}{2}$ in (3.5 cm) below navel. Let your concentration float here and if distracting thoughts arise, bring your concentration back to this area.

Physical effects Good for sufferers of neurasthenia, high blood pressure, emphysema and heart disease. It also puts emphasis on control of mind in order to achieve the quiet state.

The following chart is a specially designed schedule for convalescent patients interested in practicing qiangzhuang gong.

QIANGZHUANG GONG PRACTICING SCHEDULE

STAGE	First stage (1st week)	Second stage (2nd–4th week)	Third stage (After 4th week)
POSTURE	Sitting upright	Sitting cross-legged	Sitting or standing
BREATHING	Natural breathing	Deep abdominal breathing	Deep abdominal breathing
MIND CONTROL	Counting method	Natural method	Concentration on lower abdomen
FREQUENCY AND DURATION	3–4 times a day; each 15–20 minutes	3–4 times a day; each 30 minutes	3–4 times a day; each 30–45 minutes
POINTS TO REMEMBER	Keep posture correct. Breathing should be fine, even and steady. Dispel distracting thoughts.	Breathing should be longer, deeper and reaching down to area of lower abdomen. Begin to attain quiet state. Concentration should be easier.	Breathing should be fine, deep, long, slow, even, steady and unhurried. Achieve quiet state. Body should feel better and be growing stronger.

NEIYANG GONG (INNER GROWTH)

Neiyang gong can be done lying on the side, lying on the back or sitting upright.

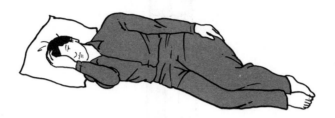

Lying on the side *Lie on right side, bend forward slightly and keep right hand on pillow about 2 in (5 cm) from the head with palm up. Rest left arm on hip with palm down and keep legs bent.*

Lying on the back *Lie down on back with a large, soft pillow under head and shoulders. Relax arms and legs, close eyes lightly and close mouth with upper and lower teeth touching each other and tip of tongue resting behind upper teeth.*

Sitting upright *Sit upright on a flat stool with feet firmly on the ground. Keep legs separate, but parallel and shoulder-width apart;*

keep torso upright, hands on thighs, elbows naturally bent, head and spine straight, chin in, shoulders relaxed, eyes and mouth lightly closed and tip of tongue resting behind upper teeth.

Breathing *Breathe through nose; use abdominal breathing method, but pause in between breaths while silently reciting certain phrases. The formula is as follows:*
Breathe in, breathe out, pause, lift tongue and silently recite certain phrases, drop tongue, breathe in and breathe out. When pausing do not hold breath, but concentrate on lower abdomen and do not block air in upper abdomen or throat. The length

of pause can be extended gradually and it can be controlled by the number of words you silently recite. One word should be recited per second and an average phrase is between three and seven words; therefore each pause will last about three to seven seconds. The phrases should be self-suggestive such as 'quiet is good', 'quiet and relaxation are good'.

Physical effects It is possible that pauses in abdominal breathing increase blood circulation in the abdomen and activate stomach and intestines. Reciting while breathing automatically achieves concentration.

UP AND DOWN BREATHING EXERCISE

This exercise, which requires physical movements, is included as a contrast to qigong movements, where the emphasis is on mental control.

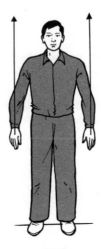

Preparation *Stand at ease with feet shoulder-width apart and body relaxed. Concentrate on movement and breathe naturally.*▶

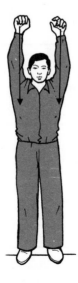

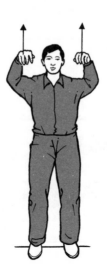

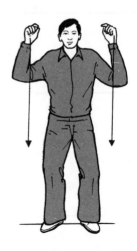

1 Bend arms slightly and raise them above head with fingers relaxed. Start breathing in as soon as you start to raise arms and

continue to do so until both arms are straight above head.
2–3 Bend knees, breathe out and start to squat. While squatting keep torso

upright and at same time lower arms in front of body and bend elbows so that hands go up.

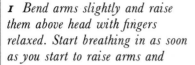

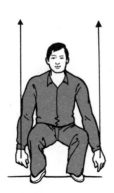

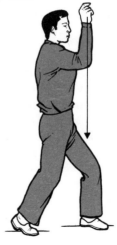

4 Bring hands down beside legs.
5 Stand up, raise arms and breathe in deeply.
Repeat exercise 10–20 times.

Variations *When standing up, raising arms and breathing in, turn body either to left or to right.*

Points to remember
● *Movements must be slow and fairly gradual.*
● *Breathing must be as fine, long and even as possible.*

Physical effects Helps to prevent high blood pressure, tracheitis and other chronic diseases. By incorporating physical movement it also enhances blood circulation, digestion, improves function of lungs and strengthens muscles in the chest and abdomen.

眼睛保健操
EYE EXERCISES

These are designed for those who spend most of their working day sitting down and doing close work. This includes writers, embroiderers, watch repairers, artists and many similar workers.

The Chinese terms for acupuncture points are used to indicate the areas to be rubbed by the hands and fingers since it is difficult to translate accurately each term into English.

PRESSING AND RUBBING ZHENG-GUANG POINTS

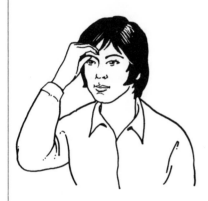 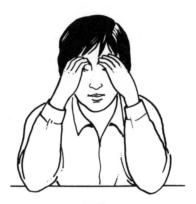 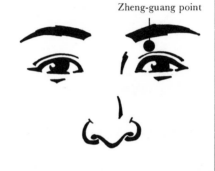

Zheng-guang point

Use both hands. Bend forefinger and middle finger and rest them on forehead. Press and rub zheng-

guang point gently under eyebrow with your thumb.
Repeat exercises eight times, each

time to a count of eight. Rub toward inside for first four; rub toward outside for last four.

SQUEEZING AND PRESSING JING-MING POINTS

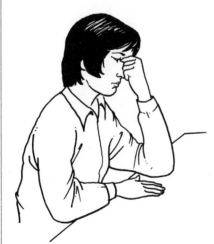 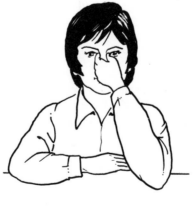 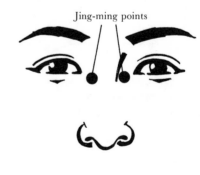

Jing-ming points

Use thumb and forefinger of either left or right hand to press and squeeze jing-ming points between

eyes and near base of nose. Press down then squeeze up.

Repeat exercise four times, each time to a count of eight, alternating the up and down movement.

眼
睛
保
健
操

PRESSING AND RUBBING SI-BAI POINTS

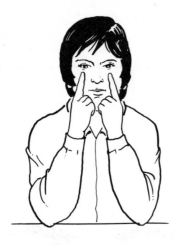 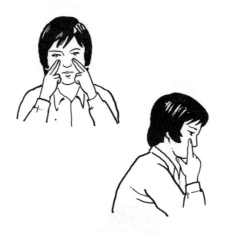 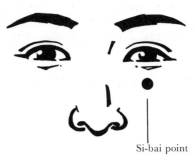

Si-bai point

Place forefinger and middle finger of each hand on each side of nose. Use thumbs to support chin. Drop middle

fingers and press and rub si-bai points just below eyes with forefingers.

Repeat exercise eight times, each time to a count of eight. Rub toward inside and outside alternately.

RUBBING AROUND THE EYE SOCKETS

Points around eye socket

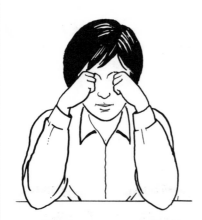 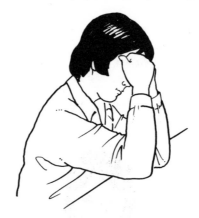 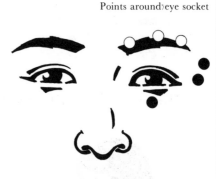

Place fists against eyebrows and thumbs against temples. Rub against eye sockets with middle joint of

forefinger, first above eye along eyebrow, then below eye. Repeat exercise eight times,

continuing to rub above and below the eye alternately to a count of eight.

MASSAGING FENG-CHI POINTS

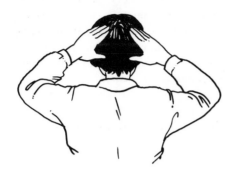

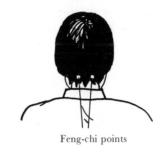

Feng-chi points

眼睛保健操

Place hands on back of head, with thumbs pressing against feng-chi points, two hollow spots under occipital bone. Massage points with thumbs. Repeat exercise four times, each time to a count of eight. *Alternate between massaging toward inside and outside.*

When you have completed the five exercises close eyes and count silently to eight, four times. Open eyes, look into distance and count to eight again four times.

Points to remember
● *When massaging, concentrate hard and do not use excessive force. Move fingers firmly but gently.*
● *Keep hands clean and locate points accurately.*
● *Do exercises regularly at least two or three times a day.*
● *Close eyes lightly during exercises and bend head slightly forward.*
● *Always keep eyes clean.*

防治按摩
SELF-MASSAGE

Some self-massage exercises require a thorough knowledge of acupuncture points. A few basic techniques which may be done lying down or sitting up are explained here and if done regularly either in the morning or at night they can greatly improve one's general health.

The main effects of self-massage are that it regulates the nervous system and helps to relieve or even prevent pain; that it builds up resistance to disease by increasing blood circulation and that it limbers up muscles and blood vessels and helps swellings to go down.

TECHNIQUES OF SELF-MASSAGE

Self-massage can be done in ten different ways and either hands or fingers can be used. Study the methods carefully and learn the Chinese terms.

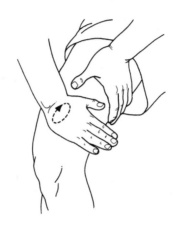

Rou *Knead skin or acupuncture points with fingers or palms.*

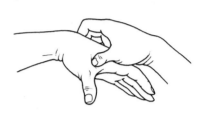

Qia *Press acupuncture points hard with fingers or finger.*

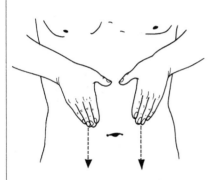

Tui *Press and push skin or acupuncture points with fingers or palms.*

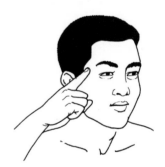

Zhi *Press acupuncture point hard with one finger.*

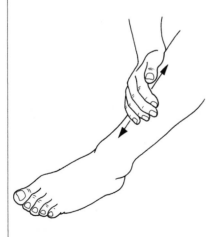

Ca *Rub skin or acupuncture points with fingers or one palm.*

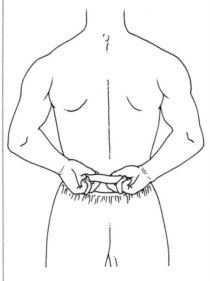

Nie *Hold muscles or ligaments with thumb, forefinger and middle finger.*

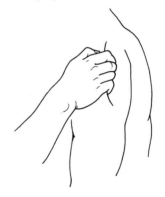

Zhua *Clutch muscles with all five fingers.*

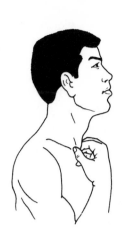

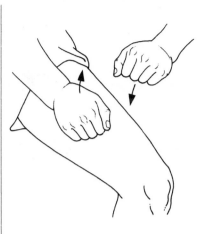

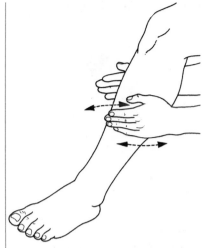

Jiu Pinch and pull up muscles with first three fingers.

Kou Pound legs or body with palms or fists.

Cuo Rub any part of body with one hand or both hands.

FIVE EXERCISES TO BE DONE LYING ON THE BED

LYING ON THE SIDE
These movements are best done in the order given here.

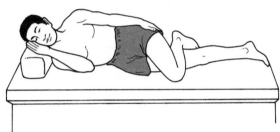

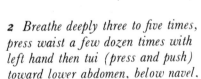

1 Lie on right side, bend right arm and hold right side of face with right hand; rest left arm on left side and keeping right leg straight, bend left knee.

2 Breathe deeply three to five times, press waist a few dozen times with left hand then tui (press and push) toward lower abdomen, below navel.

a few dozen times, then rou (knead) around navel a few dozen times.

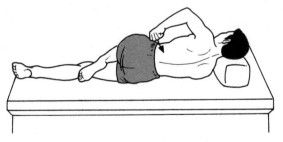

3 Tui, rou and kou (pound) back part of waist with base of left palm a few dozen times.
Repeat exercise, but lie on left side.

Physical effects Stimulates large and small intestines, bladder and kidneys and also helps to prevent difficulty in urinating and relieves constipation.

LYING ON THE STOMACH

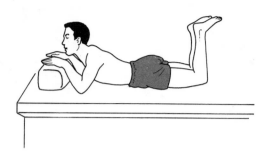
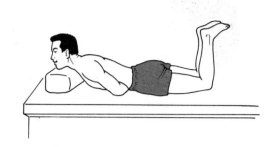

1 *Lie on stomach, head up, place hands on pillow and bend legs. Breathe deeply three to five times.*

2 *Place hands, palms up, under stomach and cushion upper abdomen, navel and lower abdomen; breathe*

deeply three to five times in each position.

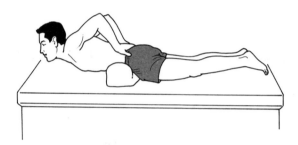

3 *Cushion abdomen with pillow and tui and rou (massage and knead) small of back a few dozen times with both hands.*

Physical effects Regularizes functions of internal organs.

LYING ON THE BACK

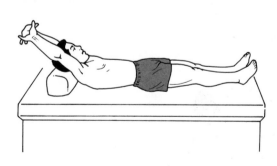
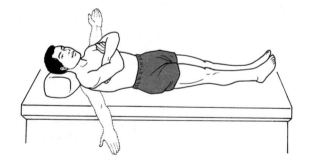

Preparation *Lie on back with arms and legs straight and breathe deeply three to five times.*
1 *Lift arms sideways above head,*

join hands with fingers interlocked and palms facing out. Breathe deeply three to five times and return arms to side.

2 *Stretch arms to side and breathe in; cross arms in front of chest and breathe out. Repeat movement three to five times.*

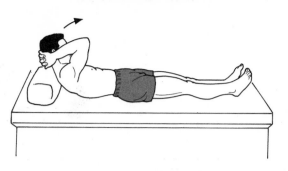

3 *Hold back of head with fingers interlocked and bend head forward so that chin touches breastbone.*

Remain in this position for a moment then return head to pillow.

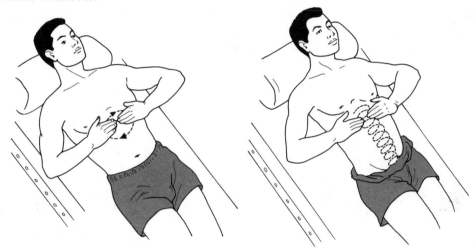

4 *Using four fingers of both hands, rou (knead) pit of stomach clockwise 20 to 30 times.*

5 *Rou (knead) intestines: using four fingers of both hands rub in small circles from pit of stomach*

downward to area below navel 20 to 30 times.

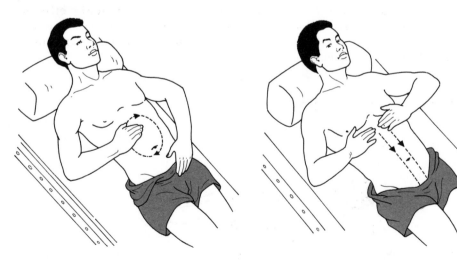

6 *Rou (knead) liver and gallbladder: place left hand on left hipbone and rub abdomen area clockwise with right hand 20 to 30 times.*

7 *Using four fingers of both hands press and push down the area between pit of stomach and pubic bones 20 to 30 times.*

Physical effects Invigorates function of spleen, stomach, liver and gallbladder and also aids digestion, relaxes bowels, prevents wind and stops hiccups.

防治按摩

BENDING LIMBS

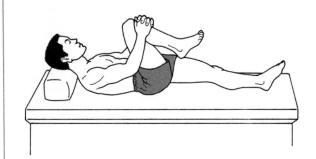

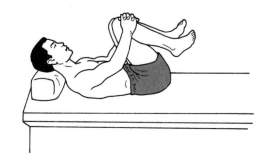

Preparation *Lie on back.*
1 Breathe deeply, bend right knee and press it close to chest with both

hands. Repeat movement with left leg and then repeat again three to five times with each leg.

2 Bend both knees and press them close to chest with both hands.

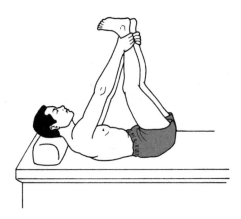

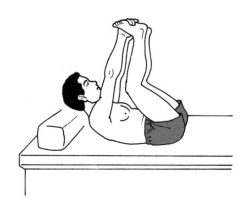

3 Bend hips and knees, hold ankles and straighten legs as much as possible.
4 Bend hips and knees, hold soles

of feet from inside and raise upper body. Remain in this position for a moment then repeat movement three to five times.

Physical effects Stimulates blood circulation and relaxes muscles and joints.

LYING CUSHIONED ON THE BACK

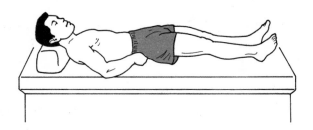

Preparation *Lie on back using fists to cushion back.*

1 Cushion sides of waist with fists and breathe deeply three to five times.

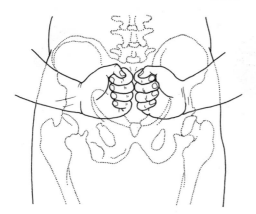

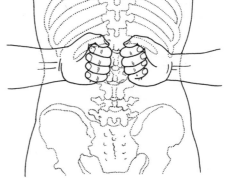

防治按摩

2 *Cushion sacrum, just below waist, with fists and breathe deeply three to five times.*
3 *Cushion end of spine with fists*

and breathe deeply three to five times.
4 *Cushion vertebrae with fists and breathe deeply three to five times.*

Physical effects Improves function of internal organs.

TWELVE EXERCISES TO BE DONE SITTING ON THE BED

These exercises should be done at night or in the morning.
Any or all of the twelve may be practiced.

HEAD AND FACE

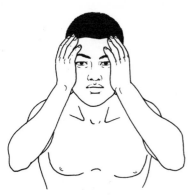

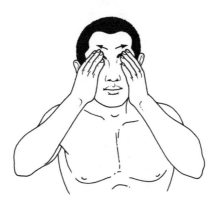

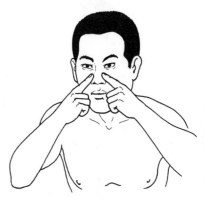

1 *Cuo (rub) palms until warm. Dry wash (rub) face until it is hot.*

2 *Tui (press and push) eyebrows and eye sockets.*

3 *Tui (press and push) both sides of nose with forefingers.*

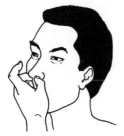

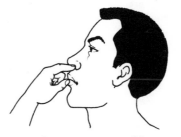

4 *Qia (press or pinch hard) nasal septum and upper lip with thumb and forefinger.*

Repeat each movement a few dozen times.

5 *Close mouth and clench teeth 20 to 30 times; swallow hard.*▶

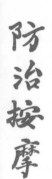

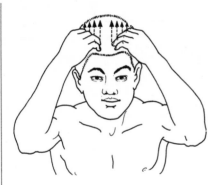

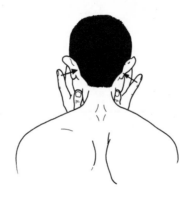

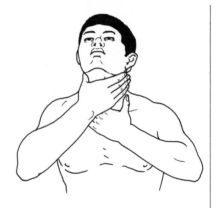

6 *Comb scalp with fingers from forehead down to nape of neck.*

7 *Press lower ears forward with middle fingers then tap back of ear lobes with forefingers a few dozen times.*

8 *Tui and cuo (rub, massage and knead) throat, neck and nape with one or both hands a few dozen times.*

Physical effects Promotes clear eyesight, sharp hearing, improved senses and a healthy complexion.

BACKWARD GLANCE

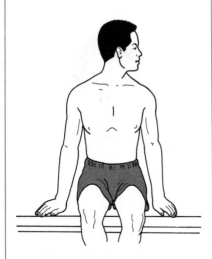

Rest hands on bed, turn head back as far as possible; follow movement with eyes, first looking up, then looking down. Alternate sides and repeat a few dozen times. The same movement can be done with arms raised to the side at shoulder level.

Physical effects Strengthens neck muscles and improves eyesight.

LOOSENING UP ELBOWS

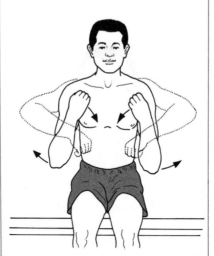

Bend forearms toward chest and move elbows forward, backward and sideways.

Physical effects Strengthens arms and elbows.

POUNDING FISTS

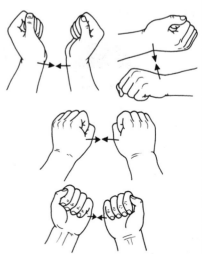

1 *Clench fists loosely and pound base of palms against each other.*
2 *Pound back of wrists against each other.*
3 *Pound thumb bones against each other.*
4 *Pound little finger bones against each other.*

Physical effects Prevents numb wrists, palms and fingers.

防治按摩

MOVING FINGERS

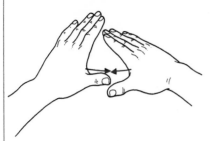

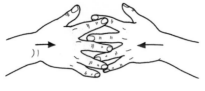

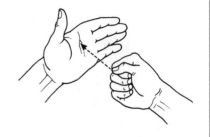

1 Spread hands out and hit them together with area between thumb and forefinger a few dozen times.

2 Repeat movement with fingers interlocked a few dozen times.

3 Clench right fist loosely and hit palm and back of left hand. Alternate hands and repeat exercise a few dozen times.

Physical effects Increases nimbleness of fingers and prevents numbness and pain.

MAKING GRABBING GESTURES

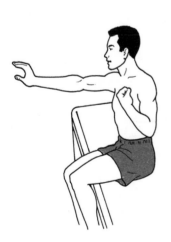

Reach out in front with right arm, place hand under arm on same side. Repeat movement a few dozen times, alternating arms and breathing deeply. This exercise can also be done with both arms reaching out at same time.

Physical effects Prevents ailments in arms and shoulders and regulates heart, lungs, liver and gallbladder.

BOW DRAWING

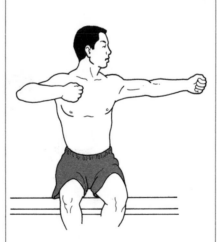

Clench fists, stretch left arm out and bend right arm into body at shoulder level as though holding a bow and arrow.
Change arms and repeat exercise a few dozen times, alternating arms and keeping eyes on arm that is stretched out and breathe deeply.

Physical effects Increases strength in shoulders and arms and expands chest.

THE SINGLE ARM LIFT

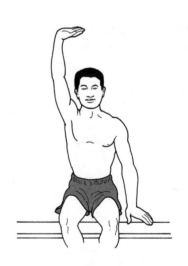

Breathe deeply and raise right arm above head, palm up and facing inward. Change arms over and repeat exercise a few dozen times.

Physical effects Strengthens arms and regulates spleen and stomach.

防治按摩

PATTING SHOULDERS AND WAIST

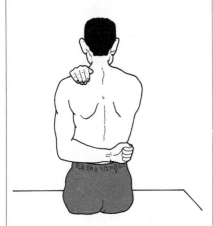

Pat left shoulder with right hand and at same time tap right side of small of back with back of left hand. Repeat exercise a few dozen times, alternating hands.

Physical effects Prevents ailments in waist and shoulders.

SWAYING

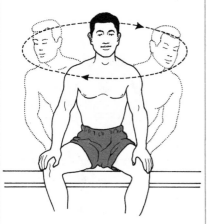

Breathe deeply, place hands on knees and sway upper body from left to right in a circle a few dozen times.

Physical effects Limbers up chest, abdomen and spinal column and also renews energy.

KICKING THE AIR

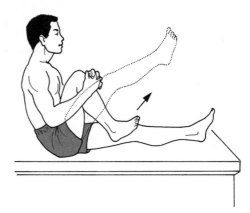

Bend one leg and clasp knee close to body. Kick up and straighten leg. Repeat exercise a few dozen times, alternating legs.

Physical effects Strengthens waist and legs and helps digestion.

PULLING TOES

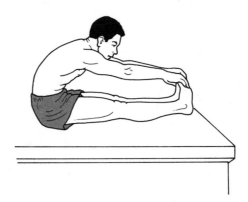

*Stretch legs, feet together, and bend forward to hold toes.
Repeat exercise a few dozen times.*

Physical effects Strengthens back, waist and kidneys.

BATHS

Baths are of great therapeutic value both to the body and to the mind. They help to stimulate the blood circulation and also to tone up the nervous system. Three completely different ways of taking a bath are described here. They are cold baths, air baths and sun baths.

COLD WATER BATHS

Become accustomed to cold water first and start by just bathing parts of your body.

FACE BATHS
Begin by washing your face with cold water when the weather is warm. After morning exercises rub your face, ears, head and neck vigorously with both palms until they are warm. Wring out a towel in cold water and use it to rub your face, ears and neck. Then take a deep breath, dip your face into cold water and breathe out in the water. Repeat many times and then rub your face, ears and neck with a wrung out, wet towel.

Physical effects Stimulates blood circulation, prevents colds and cures insomnia.

FOOT BATH
Begin by using warm water and gradually decrease the temperature of the water until it has dropped to 16° C (62° F). If the effects are good decrease the temperature of the water again until it drops to 4°C (40°F). Before taking a foot bath rub your feet until they are warm, then dip feet into water and rub them against each other. Soak your feet in the water for a few minutes, dry your feet with a towel and do some foot exercises to warm up.

Physical effects Has positive effects on whole body.

RUBBING BATH
Soak a towel in cold water, then wring out water and rub all parts of your body with the towel. Soak the towel constantly in cold water so that it retains its iciness. Dry yourself with a dry towel and put your clothes back on so as to keep warm. Remember that the time spent in the bath and the speed of rubbing depend on the temperature of the water – the colder the water, the shorter the bath and the faster the rubbing.

Physical effects This type of bath prepares one's body for cold showers.

SHOWERING AND RINSING
Before taking a cold shower exercise or rub your body with a dry towel until you are warm. For beginners the water should be about 34°–36° C (94–98° F). The temperature should then be dropped – about one degree centigrade each week – until the water is completely cold. Shower your arms and legs first, then your body and finally your face. Shower for five minutes in summer but certainly for no more than 30 seconds to a minute in winter.

SOAKING BATH
Before immersing your body from the chest down in cold water exercise to generate body warmth. Make sure that the weather is warm and gradually decrease the water temperature. Massage and rub your body with a towel while in the water and do not sit still. The time you spend soaking depends on the temperature of the water – for example, if the water is 10°C (50°F) stay in the water for only two to three minutes.

AIR BATHS

Air bathing involves exposing as much as possible of one's body to the fresh air. The physiological effects caused by the stimulation of cold air are basically the same as those caused by cold water. Chinese doctors often advise patients suffering from anaemia, hepatitis, tracheitis and heart disease to take regular air baths. They are advised to bare their bodies to the elements at every opportunity and especially in the morning.▶

WARM AIR BATHS

Take warm air baths in summer when the temperature is between 20°–30°C (70°–90°F). Massage your body or do some exercises at the same time.

COOL AIR BATHS

Take cool air baths in the autumn when the temperature is between 15°–20°C (60°–65°F). They are generally more stimulating than warm air baths and it is a good idea to do physical exercises while taking them.

COLD AIR BATHS

Do warming-up exercises before taking cold air baths and avoid windy or foggy weather. Do not expose your body to the cold air for more than five minutes and when the temperature drops to zero move indoors for cold air baths.

SUN BATHS

Sunbathing can easily be included in one's daily life – out in the fields or when playing tennis, swimming or jogging. It is best to sunbathe in the shade first so that the sun is filtered and to gradually move out into the sun. You may either sit or lie in the sun, but always remember to shield your head with a piece of cloth or an umbrella.

Begin with about five minutes of sunbathing and gradually increase the time to half an hour to an hour. Have a cold shower or go for a swim at intervals, thus combining the three elements of nature – sun, water and air.

The ideal places for sunbathing are in the mountains, where there is little dust in the air, or near a lake or river, or by the sea, where the air is moist.

Do not sunbathe when feeling dizzy or nauseous, when you have an empty stomach or immediately after a full meal. Sunbathing should also be avoided when you are feeling tired as it will only have negative effects on your body.

TABLE OF EXERCISES

This table summarizes the exercises described and illustrated in this book and explains the benefits they bring to one's physical and mental well-being. Because it is not appropriate to Wushu this is not a program of exercises. To get the most out of the table – and out of Wushu itself – note the points to remember and choose your exercise according to your own physical needs. Never exceed the limits of your physical capabilities, relax while exercising and go at your own pace.

EXERCISES	PHYSICAL EFFECTS	POINTS TO REMEMBER
Silk exercises (for adults)	Good for general well-being	Pay attention to breathing. Start exercises slowly and gradually increase the number.
First-year exercises (for babies)	Helps physical and intellectual development of children.	Do not exercise for too long – 10–20 minutes is about right. Consistency and regularity in exercising ensure the best results.
Playground exercises (for 3- to 6-year-olds)	Helps children to coordinate leg and arm movements. Ensures development of correct posture.	Do not worry if younger children do not respond so well as older children.
Farmers' exercises (for adults)	Ensures correct breathing. Strengthens muscles and bones.	All movements are independent of each other and can therefore be done in any order. Start with a few movements and gradually build up exercising program.
Coffee break exercises (for all ages)	Relieves fatigue and relaxes mind.	Concentrate on the rhythm of exercises, counting the beats as you go along.
Animal play (for adults)	Tiger play strengthens the body; deer play relaxes muscles; monkey play increases nimbleness of limbs; bear play is good for internal organs and crane play is good for lungs and helps circulation.	Relax body before starting to exercise. Start with simple exercises and gradually work through to more advanced stage. ▶

TABLE OF EXERCISES

EXERCISES	PHYSICAL EFFECTS	POINTS TO REMEMBER
Taiji shadow boxing (for all ages)	Promotes circulation and improves coordination and balance.	Be patient and learn the movements gradually. The 28 movements can be practiced as a whole or in sections.
Taiji swordplay (for all ages)	Helps to relieve stiffness in muscles and joints.	Not a vigorous kind of swordplay and is therefore also suitable for the elderly. It can be practiced alone or in groups.
The Taiji duet (for adults)	Helps to relax body and mind.	Partners should not come into direct conflict with each other.
The 18 therapies (for adults)	The first three sets of exercises help to relieve or prevent pains in the neck, shoulders, waist and legs. The second three sets of exercises help to relieve arthritis and internal disorders.	Exercise slowly and rhythmically and count the beats as you go.
Breathing exercises (for all ages)	Improves circulation and vitality.	Relax body and mind throughout and do not be impatient. Exercise in fresh air and do not breathe too deeply.
Eye exercises (for adults)	Relieves eye strain and helps preserve good vision.	Keep hands clean and do not exert too much pressure. Exercise regularly at least two or three times a day.
Self-massage (for adults)	Helps to relieve and prevent tension. Builds up resistance to disease by increasing blood circulation.	Most beneficial if done after getting up or before going to bed.
Baths (for adults)	Stimulates circulation and is generally invigorating.	Do not subject yourself to extreme temperatures at first.